Healthy, Resilient Kids: Natural Cold & Flu Survival Tips for Parents
Michael J. Vicioso, CPNP-PC

For permission requests, speaking inquiries, corporate sponsorship, bulk orders, and purchase options, email: mike@ghtkids.com

Produced by Diamond Queen.

Disclaimer:

The author in no way, shape, or form considers any of the information in this book to be a promise, guarantee, warranty, or any form of professional advice. It is intended for informational and educational purposes only. The results produced by the author, or anyone referenced in the book, are mentioned for illustration purposes only and are not intended to imply or suggest that you will have results that are similar to those in the book.

The information contained in this book is for educational and informational purposes only and is not intended as health or medical advice. Always consult a physician or other qualified health provider regarding any questions you may have about a medical condition or health objectives.

No Doctor-Patient Relationship. Although the author is a Board-Certified Pediatric Holistic Nurse Practitioner, the publication of this book does not create a doctor-patient or practitioner-patient relationship between the author and the reader. The author does not know your child's specific medical history, allergies, or needs.

Limitation of Liability. The author and publisher specifically disclaim any liability, loss, or risk, personal or otherwise, that is incurred as a consequence, directly or indirectly, of the use and application of any of the contents of this book. The strategies, supplements, and remedies discussed in this book may not be suitable for everyone.

Emergency Situations. If you think you or your child may have a medical emergency, call your doctor, go to the emergency department, or call 911 immediately.

ISBN: 979-8-9947754-0-0 (Paperback)
ISBN: 979-8-9947754-2-4 (Hardcover)
ISBN: 979-8-9947754-1-7 (EPUB)

Reviews & Testimonials

"I'm a mom of three, and we've been coming to see Mike since 2016. This book captures Mike's health philosophy using natural remedies, which aligns with our family's values. The book is easy to read for busy parents and includes go-to action tips we can implement quickly during flu and cold season. Over the years, our children's health has improved tremendously through Mike's guidance. We're grateful to Mike and his team for taking such good care of our family."

— Dr. Izdihar Jamil, Ph.D., Bestselling Author of *Speak With Influence*, TEDx Curator, and Mom of 3

"We started seeing Mike in 2013 and consider him a trusted partner in our children's healthcare journey! He always provides sound advice, while listening with an empathetic ear. His practice utilizes a balanced blend of conventional and holistic medicine, which is something I appreciate as an integrative pharmacist myself. This book encapsulates the best of Mike's wisdom, with a plethora of practical tips to guide any worried parent during cold and flu season. Mike and his staff truly go above and beyond in supporting our children…growing healthy together!

Dr. Christine Scott, Pharm D and mother of three healthy and happy children

"Chapter 2 provides practical, physiologically grounded insights into how the body responds to fever and illness. The discussion around circadian rhythm, immune response patterns, hydration, and temperature regulation offers parents a clearer understanding of what is happening during a fever and how to respond thoughtfully and appropriately."

Nancy Taschner
Nurse practitioner at GHT

HEALTHY, RESILIENT KIDS

Natural Cold and Flu Survival
Tips for Parents

Michael J. Vicioso, CPNP

Table of Contents

INTRODUCTION

WHY I WROTE THIS (AND WHY YOU'RE DOING BETTER THAN YOU THINK)

If you're reading this book at 2 a.m. with a sick child in the next room, I want you to know something: the fact that you're here, searching for answers, means you're already doing a great job.

I see parents like you every single day in my practice. They walk in exhausted, apologetic, second-guessing every decision they've made. "I'm probably just being one of those parents," they'll say, as if caring deeply about their child's health is somehow embarrassing. It's a moment any caregiver would recognize.

Let me tell you what I see: I see a parent who hasn't slept more than four hours, who's been tracking temperatures, monitoring symptoms, and going down Google rabbit holes while their child sleeps fitfully in the next room. You've got Instagram saying one thing, your mother-in-law saying another, and a dozen articles that all seem to contradict the one you read five minutes ago.

I see someone drowning in information but starving for clarity.

That's why I wrote this book. In these pages, you'll find clear, actionable steps for common situations to help you feel more confident. It's about cutting through the chaos and providing reassurance that you're doing better than you might think.

The question usually comes at the end of an appointment, just as I'm reaching for the door handle. The parent—exhausted, defeated—will hesitate and then just say it: "He's been sick three times this month. Is his immune system broken?"

What they're really asking is: Am I failing as a parent? Is there something I should be doing differently? Why does everyone else's kid seem fine while mine is always sick?

Here's what I tell them: that knot in your stomach isn't paranoia. It's what happens when you love someone small and vulnerable who can't tell you where it hurts. Every caring parent feels this way sometimes, and it's perfectly normal to worry. But that knot doesn't mean something is wrong with your child. More often than not, it means everything is working exactly as it should.

What I want to give you is something different: clarity. The kind of calm, evidence-based guidance that comes from someone who's spent eight years in a Level 1 trauma center ER, opened his own holistic pediatric practice, and raised four kids without a single hospitalization for illness.

Not because we got lucky. Because we knew what to do—and more importantly, what not to do.

THE KID WHO KNEW TOO MUCH

I grew up in a house where health wasn't a hobby—it was the air we breathed.

My dad was a physician trained in the Dominican Republic who did his residency in New York, then settled in California, where I was born. My mom was a registered nurse. Both of them were in healthcare, but more than that, they were obsessed with it. Not the "take this pill and feel better" version of medicine. The deeper kind—the "how do we actually build health" kind.

Every year, my dad would go to these big conferences in San Francisco. This was the 1970s, when the idea that diet and exercise could prevent disease was revolutionary. He'd come home with notebooks full of information that sounded like science fiction to most people.

I remember one conversation in particular. I must have been eight or nine years old. My dad was in the kitchen, cooking dinner as he always did, and I was sitting at the table doing homework.

"Dad, how come we're not having spaghetti?" I asked.

He didn't even look up from the stove. "Oh, well, because I just went to the conference, and we learned that it's important to reduce our carbohydrates and increase our proteins. So now we're having steak and vegetables."

Just like that. No pasta. No bread. The salt shaker disappeared from the table. Juice was replaced with water. My dad would explain the "why" behind every change while he was cooking—why too much salt raised blood pressure, why high-carb diets led to obesity, why vitamin C and zinc matter for immunity.

This was 1975. Most Americans were still being told that butter was the enemy and margarine was healthy. That you needed to drink a glass of whole milk with every meal,—that cholesterol from eggs would kill you.

My dad knew better. And he made sure we did too.

So when I'd go to a friend's house for dinner, I'd sit there staring at a table loaded with pasta, garlic bread, and salt shakers, and I'd politely take a small serving of pasta, skip the bread entirely, and refuse the salt.

"What's wrong with you?" my friends would ask. "Why aren't you eating more?"

"This isn't good for me," I'd say. "This is gonna make me fat and unhealthy."

They looked at me like I was from another planet.

My friends called me “Doc.”[2] Sometimes it was affectionate. Sometimes it wasn't. I was a ten-year-old kid who couldn't stop talking about health, who brought vitamin C supplements to sleepovers, who'd lecture people about sugar content in juice boxes.

I couldn't help myself. I wanted everyone to know there was a better way to feel.

THE “SYSTEM” VS. THE REALITY

That drive eventually pushed me into medicine. I went to nursing school in LA County—the hotbed of everything that happens in the world medically. I saw Legionnaire's’ disease. I saw rare tropical infections. I saw cases that would end up in textbooks.

I worked at Children's Hospital Los Angeles for eight years in the emergency department. It's a Level 1 trauma center—the place where the worst cases go. I saw children at their most vulnerable, and I learned how to save lives in situations where seconds mattered.

I went back to school, got my board-certified pediatric nurse practitioner degree from California State University, Long Beach, and became a hospitalist at CHOC (Children's Hospital of Orange County), admitting and discharging patients.

But the more I worked in the system, the more limited I felt.

That's when I made a deliberate choice. While completing my training at CSU Long Beach, I sought out pediatricians who specialized in alternative and complementary medicine. I wanted to learn both worlds—traditional pediatrics and CAM—so I could offer families real options, not just prescriptions.

Don't get me wrong—I believe in evidence-based medicine. Hospitals follow protocols that save lives, and I'm grateful for that. But there's little room for customization. No room for considering the individual child, the individual family, the cultural practices that matter to them. Hospital systems are giants,-slow to change. The old adage is that it takes 50 years for research findings to reach actual practice. I wanted to shorten that time and get the latest information to my patients, so they would be aware and have options.

I'd see a family from Malaysia walk in, and I'd know they were comfortable using coconut water for hydration. It's what they'd always used. It's safe, it works, it's full of electrolytes. But could I order coconut water from the hospital kitchen? No. It wasn't in the system. So I'd have to hand them a bottle of artificially flavored Pedialyte instead.

I'd want to suggest warm garlic oil for an earache—something that's been used safely for generations, something that actually works—but it wasn't in the hospital formulary. It wasn't "approved." So I couldn't mention it.

I had all this knowledge—from my training, from my father, from years of practice—and I couldn't use it.

The only way I could figure out how to share what I knew was to open my own practice.

In 2013, literally one year after getting my nurse practitioner degree, I partnered with another provider and opened a practice in Long Beach. It was there, finally, that I got to teach people what I'd learned from my parents, from my training, and from caring for my own children—to provide care that incorporated all aspects of health: traditional medicine, folk medicine, holistic approaches, Eastern and Western modalities, all together in one place.

It was something new. Something Long Beach hadn't seen before. And it gave me a foothold to do what I'd wanted to do my entire life: help families build health, not just treat disease.

From a Dad Who's Been There

I'm not just coming at this as a provider. I'm a father of four—Joseph, Emily, Genevieve, and Jessica. I've lived through the long nights. I've had the same panicked thoughts you've had.

Bringing my knowledge into my own family was humbling. You think having medical training makes parenting easier? It doesn't. If anything, it makes you second-guess yourself more.

You're confronted by competing theories. Outdated advice. Pressure from well-meaning people who think they know better.

We'd go to wellness visits, and the pediatrician would give us what felt like outdated advice: Feed your baby full-fat milk. Use formula if breastfeeding is hard. Here are antibiotics for that runny nose.

And I'd sit there, nodding my head, saying, "Yes, doctor, whatever you say."

Then I'd go home and do what I knew was right.

We didn't feed our kids full-fat milk. We knew it contributed to atherosclerosis—hardening of the arteries—later in life. We used non-fat or low-fat milk, and only in small amounts with cereals or smoothies.

When the kids got sick, doctors would prescribe antibiotics immediately. "Your kid has a runny nose, cough, and fever? Here's amoxicillin."

No. I knew better. Most of those illnesses were viral. Antibiotics don't kill viruses. So instead, we'd support the body with hydration, nutrition, and rest. We'd let the immune system do its job.

My kids struggled through illnesses like every other child, but we were intentional about not jumping to medications. Over time, I saw what I now see in my patients: when the basics are in place—good hydration, solid nutrition, natural light, plenty of movement—and medications are used thoughtfully, kids usually recover faster and need fewer interventions.

I can't think of a single time—knock on wood—when I had to admit any of my children to the hospital for illness. Sure, there were a few times they needed antibiotics for a serious ear infection or possible pneumonia. But those times were rare.

They got sick often, just like every other kid. But nothing required significant medical intervention. Because we gave their bodies what they needed to heal: hydration, sleep, good nutrition, and time.

And that's another reason I opened my practice—to share that knowledge with other families. To give them permission to trust their instincts. To teach them when to worry and when to let the body do its work.

What This Book Will Give You

I'm not going to promise you that your child will never get sick. That would be a lie, and frankly, it wouldn't even be good for them. (We'll talk about why in Chapter 1.)

What I will give you is this:

By the end of this book, you'll have:

- A clear picture of what's normal illness and what's a red flag.
- Simple, step-by-step plans for the most common sick-kid situations.
- Everyday habits that quietly build your child's immune resilience.
- Language you can use with your pediatric provider so you feel like a partner, not a bystander.

This book will teach you how to raise healthy, resilient kids—not kids who never get sick, but kids whose bodies know how to fight, recover, and come back stronger.

You'll learn which symptoms you can manage at home and which ones require a call to your provider. You'll spend less time spiraling through midnight searches because you'll already know what to do.

And most importantly, you'll feel less like you're failing and more like you're leading.

I know you've seen the Instagram posts from that influencer mom whose kids "never get sick." (Spoiler: They do. She just doesn't post about it.) I know you've scrolled through parenting forums at 3 a.m., reading horror stories that made your anxiety spike. I know you've compared yourself to other parents and felt like you're coming up short.

Stop.

The fact that you're here, reading this book, researching, trying to do right by your child—that already makes you a great parent. You're not looking for shortcuts. You're looking for real answers.

That's exactly what I'm going to give you.

How to Use This Book

Don't feel like you have to read this cover-to-cover tonight. Think of it as a friend who happens to be a medical provider—someone you wish you could text or message at any time when you're not sure what to do.

Part 1 is your "right now" guide. If your child is coughing, running a fever, or pulling at their ears, go here first. These chapters walk you through the most common symptoms and what to do about them—without panic, without an unnecessary ER visit, and without second-guessing yourself.

Part 2 is the long game. This is about building health before illness strikes—nutrition, sleep, managing stress (yes, even kids have stress), and creating an environment where their immune systems can thrive.

Part 3 is your day-to-day toolkit on how to prepare for flu season and other high-risk times of year. What to stock in your medicine cabinet. How to adjust routines around school and activities. How to make the immune-supportive food and drink your kids will actually take.

And here's something important: make sure you read all the way to the end. In the bonus section, you'll find a Quick-Action Checklist for those middle-of-the-night moments when you just need to know what to do right now. You'll also find family-friendly recipes that support immunity—food your kids will actually eat, not kale smoothies they'll refuse.

Here's what you'll know by the end:

- Why that turtle in your child's bedroom might be causing chronic diarrhea (Chapter 6).
- How to safely bring down a 102°F fever without immediately reaching for medication (Chapter 2).
- Why your high schooler sometimes gets sicker than your kindergartener—and what to do about it (Chapter 7).
- How to calculate a practical daily water target for your child (Chapter 7).
- When elderberry actually helps and when it doesn't (Chapter 7: timing is everything).
- How moving a video game console out of the bedroom can reverse early prediabetic changes (Chapter 5).

These are the tools I wish I could hand to every parent who's awake at 2 a.m. wondering what to do.

My Hope for You

My hope for you is simple: I hope that this book makes you feel less alone at 2 a.m., more confident in your gut, and more trusting of your child's ability to heal.

By the time you finish this book, you'll understand how your child's body actually works. You'll know when to intervene and when to let the body do its job. I want you to have the same knowledge I had growing up—the kind my dad and grandparents gave me whenever I got sick. I happened to have a doctor in the house. This book gives you that same advantage—the basic knowledge to care for your child at home when they have a normal cold or flu, the illnesses that resolve on their own with guidance.

But more than that, my hope is that you'll raise healthy, resilient kids—children whose immune systems are strong not because they never get sick, but because they know how to recover. Kids who grow into adults with robust health, who don't burn out in their 30s, who live longer, healthier, happier lives because you laid the foundation now.

The work you're doing today—the late nights, the careful choices, the patience when everyone else is telling you to 'just give them antibiotics'—that work compounds. It doesn't just get your child through this cold. It sets them up for decades of vitality.

Parenting is hard enough without every cold feeling like a final exam. You're not failing because your kid caught a virus. You're not failing because you Googled symptoms at midnight. You're not failing because you're reading this book right now, desperately hoping for clarity. In this book, I will provide clear guidelines on when to let the body do its work and when to seek medical help. This way, you can feel reassured that you're making the right decisions for your child's health.

You're doing exactly what you should be doing: seeking knowledge. Asking questions. Trying to understand.

The truth is, your child's immune system isn't broken. It's learning. It's building strength with every runny nose, every cough, every fever. And you're learning too—how to support them, how to trust the process, how to tell the difference between "this is normal" and "we need help."

This book won't replace your pediatrician. I'm not trying to. We pediatric providers are here to support you through growth and development, to catch problems you might not see, to use our medical training to identify issues early. That's not replaceable by a book or even by AI.

But what this book can do is fill the gap—the space between the doctor's office and your kitchen at 2 a.m. It can give you the confidence to manage common illnesses at home. It can teach you the fundamentals of building health, not just treating symptoms.

It can give you permission to trust yourself.

You already care enough to be reading this. You're already staying up late, asking questions, putting in the work. That means you're already doing a great job.

Now let's make sure you have the tools to back up that instinct.

Before I give you a single tool—before I tell you what to do about that fever at 2 a.m.—you need to understand something fundamental that will change how you see every runny nose, every cough, every illness for the rest of your parenting life:

Your child is not sick because their immune system is broken.

They're sick because it's working.

Once you understand that, everything else clicks into place. The anxiety shuts down. The guilt evaporates. And suddenly, that fever doesn't feel like a crisis anymore—it feels like progress.

In Chapter 1, we'll start with exactly why kids get sick so often—and why that's more reassuring than it sounds.

CHAPTER 1

WHY KIDS GET SICK

If you're reading this, you're probably in one of two places: wiping a runny nose for the third time this hour, or bracing yourself for the inevitable flu season email from your child's school. For many families, childhood feels like a revolving door of illness: runny noses, coughs, fevers, and only brief stretches of health before the next thing. For parents, it's exhausting. It means missed work, broken sleep, and a quiet question that lingers in the background: Is my child's immune system weak? Am I doing something wrong?

Now picture this: it's 2 a.m. again. You're hovering over a small, hot forehead, counting breaths, whispering, "You okay, baby?" and wondering how it is even possible for someone so tiny to have this many colds in one year. If that's you, this book is for you. Millions of parents are in this same season, quietly doing night-shift duty beside a child's bed, feeling worried, depleted, and a little alone. This chapter is meant to sit on your nightstand—right after the introduction—and make those moments feel less scary and less lonely.

Your child is not broken. Your parenting is not failing. What you are living through, as messy, exhausting, and scary as it feels, is what a healthy immune system looks like when it's still under construction.

In this book, *Healthy, Resilient Kids,* we'll explore how children get sick and, more importantly, how you can support them naturally, so their immune system learns, strengthens, and recovers faster.

The goal is to give you the confidence to handle illness with calm and clarity.

To move through these years with confidence, we need to rethink illness. We need to understand the difference between being exposed to germs and becoming infected, how a child's immune system learns over time, and what everyday factors tip the scales from exposed to infected.

The Hidden Job of Childhood

From the outside, childhood looks like playdates, bedtime stories, and grass-stained knees. Inside your child's body, something much bigger is happening. Every time your child gets sick, their immune system is learning: this is what this virus looks like. This is how we fight it. Next time, we'll be faster.

To you, it feels like one more week of wiping noses, changing damp pillowcases, and rearranging work meetings. To your child's body, it's a training camp. If you could zoom in, you'd see an army of tiny cells waking up, racing down microscopic hallways, and taking notes. That runny nose, that fever, that cranky, clingy day on the couch—this is your child's body building a memory bank that will protect them for decades.

You are not just getting through another cold. You are watching the immune system grow up, even on the days it feels less like heroism and more like wiping the same little nose for the hundredth time.

Changing How We Think About Illness

This shift didn't come easily for me either. Like many parents, I watched my own kids get sick again and again and wondered if I was doing enough. Over time, I noticed something important: when the basics were in place—hydration, good food, rest, and calm support—they didn't just get better. They got better faster. Their illnesses became shorter, milder, and more predictable. These simple, natural fundamentals are some of the most powerful tools you have for helping children build lasting immunity and resilience—and for feeling that what you're doing really matters.

When I first opened my practice, parents came in with the same concern: "My child is sick all the time. Every month it's something new." A runny nose, a cough, a fever, vomiting, diarrhea. I would walk them through how immunity develops and why exposure, especially as kids get older, is part of building a healthy immune system. One of the most important mindset shifts is letting go of the belief that illness itself is always bad.

We're not talking about newborns here, but about toddlers and school-age children who are out in the world—at the park, at school, at Disneyland, at the library, at the beach—being exposed to other people and their environments. Sometimes, they bring something home. And sometimes, they get sick. That process, when appropriately supported, is how resilience is built.

In my practice, I sometimes joke with parents: if I see a one- or two-year-old who has never been sick, I start asking questions. Are they getting out? Are they around other kids? Are they exploring? A complete lack of illness in an older infant or toddler often means very little exposure, not perfect health. Kids need reasonable exposure to build a competent immune system.

How Germs Travel: From Exposure to Infection

Before we can feel calmer about illness, it helps to understand how germs get from one person to another. Viruses are like invisible hitchhikers: they cannot move on their own, so they need a ride from one person to another. You can be exposed to a virus when it lands on your hands or in your nose. You only become infected if it gets past your body's defenses and starts multiplying.

There are three main roads they use:

- Direct contact: One person touches another—holding hands, wiping a nose, comforting a crying child.

- Respiratory droplets: Tiny drops from coughs, sneezes, and even loud talking that can land on nearby people or surfaces.
- Contaminated surfaces (fomites): Germs land on desks, toys, doorknobs, markers, and then catch a ride when someone else touches those objects and then their own face.

If you've ever watched a preschooler in slow motion, touching the play kitchen, rubbing their eyes, grabbing a shared crayon, then sticking their fingers in their mouth, you've basically watched a virus take an Uber.

THE SCHOOL PETRI DISH

There are few places better designed for viral spread than a classroom. Many children sit close together, share supplies, and are still learning basic hygiene.

In a classroom, a sneeze is not just a sound; it is a dispersal event. Droplets land on desks, toys, markers, and doorknobs. Another child touches that surface, rubs their eye, eats a snack, and the virus finds a new host. This isn't a failure of schools or parents. It's the reality of joining group environments.

When a child first enters daycare, preschool, or kindergarten, many parents notice exactly what one mom described: "Every month, there's always something —a runny nose, cough, a new bug— even when my child is only going one day a week." Even limited time in a group setting can introduce a whole new set of viruses their body hasn't met yet. That is the power of exposure.

THE PING-PONG INSIDE YOUR HOME

Once a virus hitchhikes home on your child, it enters the family ecosystem. Maybe this sounds familiar:

- Week 1: Your 6-year-old comes home with a runny nose and a low-grade fever.
- Week 2: Just as the 6-year-old is better, the toddler starts vomiting and has diarrhea.
- Week 3: The toddler is finally back to normal, and now you feel awful.

Families share bathrooms, kitchen counters, towels, couches, hugs, and kisses. Because of this close, constant contact, the viral load—the amount of virus everyone is exposed to— can be even higher at home than in public spaces. A crucial fact: many children are often contagious before they look sick. By the time your child wakes up with a fever, they may have been spreading the virus for a day already. If you feel like illness just explodes in your house out of nowhere, you are not imagining it—that is often how viruses actually work.

Every family with more than one child recognizes the cascading effect. The older child brings something home from school, passes it to the younger sibling, and the younger one seems to get sick earlier in life but often handles that same bug more smoothly as they grow. Over time, those earlier exposures give younger siblings a head start in building immune memory. It becomes a kind of domino effect of immunity.

With the right care and fundamentals, though, the ping-pong effect doesn't have to feel endless. Hydration, nutrition, rest, and calm support can help make each illness episode shorter, milder, and easier to manage. Over time, both the frequency and severity of illness decrease.

THE PATTERN DOCTORS EXPECT

Here is another piece that helps parents relax: there is a very common viral pattern we see over and over.

Doctors often see a predictable sequence:

- About 3 days of symptoms building.
- Peak misery around days 3-5.
- Another 7-10 days of gradual recovery, sometimes with a lingering cough or fatigue.

A "simple" viral illness often has 3 days coming on, 3-5 days of feeling the worst, and about 10 days of recovery, sometimes with another week before your child seems completely back to themselves. We recognize this as a typical viral course, especially in younger kids who are still building immunity.

During the early school years, many children experience multiple viral illnesses per year before their immune systems mature enough to respond more quickly. When parents understand this, fear can start to give way to confidence. You can recognize a typical illness pattern and know what to expect next.

There are times when I do worry as a pediatrician—over things like trouble breathing, unusual sleepiness, signs of dehydration, or a child who seems to be getting worse instead of better—and later chapters will walk you through those red flags in detail, so you are not guessing in the dark. Some illnesses are a normal part of childhood; getting out into the world, within reason, gives the immune system the experience it needs to grow stronger over time.

Inexperienced, Not Weak: How Immunity Grows

Here is the most crucial idea in this chapter: a child who gets sick a lot does not automatically have a weak immune system. Most often, they have an inexperienced one.

Think of your child's immune system like a library.

Innate immunity is the security guard at the door. It includes skin, stomach acid, and mucous lining in the nose and throat. It reacts quickly and in a general way to almost anything that shouldn't be there.

Adaptive immunity is the librarian. It keeps a record of every "book" (virus) it has seen. When adults meet a familiar cold virus, the librarian flips through the catalog, says "We've seen this before," and releases specific antibodies to knock it out, often before any symptoms appear.

A young child's library is mostly empty. Every virus is a brand-new book. Their body has to pause, study the invader, and build a custom defense from scratch. That process takes time and energy, and the signs of that work are what we see as illness:

- **Fever**, which raises body temperature to make it harder for viruses to survive.
- **Mucus**, which traps and flushes out germs.

In the first few years of daycare or school, it is common for a child to have many colds per year. Exhausting for parents, yes, but medically, it often means the immune system is doing its job—building the library. So if your 3-year-old seems sick every few weeks, that can still fall within the normal range, and it is always okay to talk with your pediatrician about your concerns.

BLUEPRINT AND ENVIRONMENT: WHY SOME KIDS SEEM SICKER

If all kids have immune systems, why do some seem to get sick more than others? Part of the answer lies in family traits. Some pieces of innate immunity are influenced by genetics. Members of the same family can have slight differences in things like:

- The thickness of their mucous membranes.
- The amount of natural germ-fighting proteins in their saliva.

These tiny variations can make it slightly easier or harder for germs to get a foothold in different people.

Then there is **epigenetics**, which is a big word for a simple idea: your child's genes are the basic instructions, but their environment helps decide which instructions get used. Factors such as diet, sleep, stress, and exposure to germs can influence certain genes to speak up or quiet down, without changing the DNA itself.

You can think of it like sticky notes on the instruction manual: "Read this page more." "Skip this part." "Use this only in emergencies." Genes provide the instructions; epigenetics helps decide which instructions are read, and how often. Over time, that can shape how strong, fast, or calm the immune response is.

This is the bridge between your child's blueprint and their everyday life. Genetics sets the potential. Environment—including stress, nutrition, sleep, and exposure—shapes how that potential is used. The good news is that while you cannot rewrite your child's genes, you can influence the environment they grow up in. There is real, practical power in the ordinary things you do every day.

A Real Boy, a Real Year, and Many Illnesses

During my pediatric training with a pediatrician in Orange County, we followed one boy through his first year of school. His story could easily be your child's.

- Summer visit: He came in healthy—just needed school forms filled out and signed. We talked about hydration and sun safety. His mom laughed and said she hoped she wouldn't have to be at the doctor's office too often once school started.

- Mid-September: A few weeks after kindergarten began, he was back with a runny nose, cough, and fever. Classic cold. We showed his parents how to support him and said, "Once he's been fever-free for 24 hours, he can go back to school."

- October: He returned with vomiting, diarrhea, and a rash. Likely viral gastroenteritis. We focused on hydration, simple foods like bananas, and watching for dehydration. When he'd been fever-free and free of vomiting and diarrhea for 24 hours, he returned to class.

By Thanksgiving, there was another illness. This pattern continued—cold after cold, stomach bug after stomach bug—through the fall and winter. By spring, his mom joked she should have a parking spot with her name on it in front of the clinic. By the end of that school year, we had counted **17** separate viral illnesses.

That didn't mean something was wrong. It meant his immune system had entered a completely new environment. New kids, new viruses, new exposures. Each illness introduced his body to something unfamiliar. Each recovery built immune memory. To his parents, it felt never-ending. To us, as pediatricians, it was very common for a child's first year in a large-group setting. Each illness was not a sign of failure. Each one was a lesson.

His immune system:

- Studied the new virus.
- Built the right tools to fight it.
- Filed those tools in his immune library for next time.

As he got older, he became sick less often. When he did, he recovered more quickly. That is what immune resilience looks like over time, and it is where your child is headed as well.

COMMON TRIGGERS: WHAT TIPS THE SCALES

A virus always needs a host, but the state of that host—your child's overall condition—matters a lot. You cannot control every virus they meet, but you can influence the terrain the virus lands on. Stress, sugar, and environment can quietly make it easier or harder for your child to handle everyday germs.

1. Stress: The Silent Underminer

We often assume children's lives are simple and carefree, but many kids carry real stress: schoolwork and tests, friendship struggles or bullying, and busy, unpredictable schedules at home. When stress sticks around, the body produces more cortisol, a stress hormone. In short bursts, cortisol can be helpful. But when levels remain high for an extended period, cortisol can suppress the immune response, making it harder for the body to fight off invaders. A chronically stressed child is more vulnerable.

Supporting emotional health, connection, predictable routines, and genuine downtime is not just good for behavior and mood; it directly supports immunity. If you've ever watched your child fall sick right after a tough week at school or a big family change, you've seen this connection in real life.

2. The Sugar Dip: A Window of Vulnerability

Diet plays a surprisingly quick role in immunity. After a big sugar surge—like consuming soda, candy, or a dessert-heavy party—specific white blood cells called neutrophils do not work as well for several hours. Neutrophils are like the Pac-Man of the immune system: they chase and swallow invading bacteria. When blood sugar spikes, their ability to do this drops temporarily, creating a small window of vulnerability when germs have an easier time getting started.

This does not mean your child can never have a treat. You don't need to eliminate sugar, but being mindful about frequency and pairing it with protein can support the immune system, especially during seasons when everyone's sick.

3. Environment: Dry Air and the Great Indoors

Several environmental factors quietly shape your child's defenses:

- Dry air: In winter, indoor heating dries out the air and the mucous membranes inside the nose. Usually, the nose acts like sticky flypaper, trapping viruses. When it dries and cracks, that trap fails, and viruses can slip more easily into the lungs.

- The Great Indoors: Flu season is not caused by cold weather alone. It is driven by how we behave when it is cold—we close windows, stay inside, and share the same recycled air in homes, classrooms, and offices. Germs love that.

You cannot change the season. But you can soften its impact on your child's body—and on your calendar.

YOUR EVERYDAY POWER: TINY HABITS, BIG IMPACT

If illness is part of the process, where do you fit in? What can you control? You cannot bubble-wrap your child from every virus. But you can:

- Shape the terrain inside their body.
- Build routines that quietly protect and support their immune system.
- Lower how often and how severely they get sick.

Here are simple, realistic moves that make a bigger difference than most parents realize.

QUICK TIPS PARENTS CAN USE RIGHT AWAY

Strategy	Action Step
Hydrate the nose	Run a cool-mist humidifier in your child's bedroom during dry months. A moist nose acts like a guarded gate, trapping viruses before they get deeper into the body.

Strategy	Action Step
Home arrival routine	When anyone comes home from school, daycare, or work: shoes off, backpack down, then wash hands before touching siblings, pets, food, or the couch.
Protect sleep	Treat bedtime like medicine. Create a consistent, calming routine and protect enough sleep so your child's body can release key immune messengers and repair itself overnight.
Protein before sugar	Offer snacks like apple slices with nut butter, cheese and crackers, or yogurt and nuts after school to keep blood sugar steady and support immune cells.
Teach the vampire cough	Show kids how to cough or sneeze into the crook of their elbow—like a vampire with a cape—so their hands don't become germ stamps on every surface. Even toddlers can learn this with practice and modeling.

Each of these is small on its own. Together, they gently nudge the odds in your child's favor, resulting in fewer infections, milder symptoms, and faster recoveries. You can't prevent every illness, but you can reduce how often it occurs and how severe it is. Supporting your child's sleep, nutrition, hydration, and stress gives their immune system the best environment to work naturally. These simple strategies don't require perfection; they just give your child's immune system better conditions to do what it's designed to do.

YOUR ROLE: STEWARD, NOT SUPERHERO

This book will not promise a germ-free childhood. That is neither possible nor healthy. What it will offer is something better:

- A clear picture of what is normal, even when it looks scary.
- Practical ways to support your child's body through illness.
- Tools to lower how often and how hard your child gets hit.
- A calmer, more grounded mindset for you.

You don't have to be a superhero or a medical expert. Your role is not to stop every germ. Your role is to:

- Steward your child's environment.
- Provide the fundamentals, including hydration, real food, sleep, and comfort.
- Practice and model simple habits that slow the ping-pong of illness.
- Learn when a common virus is just doing its job, and when it is time to seek help.

Understanding why children get sick provides context, but parents want to know what to do when it happens. Often, that moment begins with a fever. In the next chapter, we'll talk about what fever actually is, when it's doing its job, when to worry, and how to support it safely and naturally, so you can respond with clarity instead of panic, and confidence instead of fear.

In the chapters ahead, you will learn how to:

- Walk through fevers without spiraling into panic.
- Set up your home so viruses do not rule the calendar.
- Use small, daily choices as powerful investments in your child's long-term health.

- Spot the red flags that mean "This is not typical—we need care."

For now, as you sit beside a small bed or fold yet another pile of sick-day laundry, let this sink in: the runny nose you are wiping, the cough you are counting, the third cold since school started—they are not proof that you are failing. They are proof that your child's immune system is in session, taking notes, building memory, and becoming the resilient defender they will rely on for the rest of their life. You are not just surviving this season; you are quietly helping your child build a lifelong shield.

References

Bermick, J., & Schleiss, M. R. (2022). Epigenetic regulation of pediatric and neonatal immune responses. Pediatric Research, 91(2), 297–327. *https://doi.org/10.1038/s41390-021-01630-3*

Goenka, A., & Kollmann, T. R. (2015). Development of immunity in early life. The Journal of Infection, 71(Suppl. 1), S112–S115. *https://doi.org/10.1016/j.jinf.2015.04.027*

Gollwitzer, E. S., & Marsland, B. J. (2015). Impact of early-life exposures on immune maturation and susceptibility to disease. Trends in Immunology, 36(11), 684–696. *https://doi.org/10.1016/j.it.2015.09.009*

Hong, M., & Bhatt, D. L. (2023). On developmental programming of the immune system. Trends in Immunology, 44(11), 877–889. *https://doi.org/10.1016/j.it.2023.09.005*

Jefferson, T., Dooley, L., Ferroni, E., Al-Ansary, L. A., van Driel, M. L., Bawazeer, G. A., Jones, M. A., Hoffmann, T. C., Clark, J., Beller, E. M., Glasziou, P. P., & Conly, J. M. (2023). Physical interventions to interrupt or reduce the spread of respiratory viruses. Cochrane Database of Systematic Reviews, 2023(1), CD006207. *https://doi.org/10.1002/14651858.CD006207.pub6*

Kollmann, T. R., Kampmann, B., Mazmanian, S. K., Marchant, A., & Levy, O. (2018). Immunity in the very young: Challenges and opportunities. Immunity, 49(4), 604–618. *https://doi.org/10.1016/j.immuni.2018.08.009*

Prescott, S. L., Pawankar, R., Allen, K. J., Campbell, D. E., Sinn, J. K., Fiocchi, A., Ebisawa, M., Sampson, H. A., Beyer, K., & Lee, B. W. (2011). The influence of early environmental exposures on immune development and subsequent risk of allergic disease. Allergy, 66(5), 562–575. *https://doi.org/10.1111/j.1398-9995.2011.02620.x*

Raedler, D., & Schaub, B. (2014). Immune mechanisms and development of childhood asthma. The Lancet Respiratory Medicine, 2(3), 232–242. *https://doi.org/10.1016/S2213-2600(13)70257-4*

Zhang, X., Zhivaki, D., & Lo-Man, R. (2017). Unique aspects of the neonatal immune system. Nature Reviews Immunology, 17(8), 495–507. *https://doi.org/10.1038/nri.2017.58*

CHAPTER 2

FEVER 102°+ (THE HEAT OF THE BATTLE)

Few things spike a parent's heart rate faster than touching a child's forehead and feeling heat. The thermometer beeps, the number reads 102.5°F, and instinct kicks in: *panic. Fix it. Bring it down. Now.*

Fever is often seen as a parent's nightmare, provoking an immediate urge to act and eliminate the heat that signals something might be wrong. It's important to acknowledge that this reaction is deeply rooted in past experiences that can make fever seem like our child's enemy. This instinctual fear, or "fever phobia," pushes us to combat the very process designed to help our child's body heal.

In my clinic, I see this play out over and over. Parents arrive exhausted and scared, clutching a crumpled printout of temperatures they have checked every hour. What they remember most is the number on the screen, not how their child was actually doing in between those beeps.

In this chapter, I want to flip that script. Instead of seeing fever as a fire to extinguish, we'll look at it as the body's oven, turned up on purpose to bake out an infection. We'll walk through what's normal, what's worrisome, and what you can actually do at 2 a.m. when everyone is exhausted.

In Chapter 1, we talked about how a young immune system is not weak but inexperienced, still learning what different viruses look like and how to fight them off. Fever is one of the clearest signs that your child's immune system has recognized an invader, remembered what to do, and is actively working on it.

1. The "Fever Phobia" Reset: Treat the Child, Not the Number

First, the basics.

Viruses and bacteria do best at normal body temperature, about 98.6°F. When the immune system finds an invader, the brain's thermostat, called the hypothalamus, raises the body's temperature on purpose.

When your child's temperature climbs to around 101°F, the germs stop multiplying so quickly, and by 102°F and higher, the heat makes it harder for them to survive, while your child's infection-fighting white blood cells really kick into gear.

The Golden Rule: *treat your child, not the number on the thermometer.*

A child with a fever of 103°F who is drinking fluids, watching cartoons, and responding to you is usually less concerning than a child with a temperature of 100.5°F who is limp, pale, or not responding. The height of the fever does not always match the severity of the illness. How your child looks and acts matters more than what the thermometer says.

A story from the exam room

One afternoon, a young couple brought in their eight -month-old baby, absolutely convinced that something terrible was happening. They were from a Hispanic family that held a deeply rooted hot-cold belief: you treat heat with cold and cold with heat. To them, a child who *felt* cold as the fever was rising needed to be bundled to stay warm.

By the time they arrived, the baby looked like a tiny cocoon. He had a hood pulled tight, multiple layers of clothes, and blankets wrapped around him. Only his eyes were visible, and they were clearly miserable. When we started to undress him, his hair and clothes were drenched. He was sweating through every layer.

We took everything off, let some air reach his skin, and checked his temperature. It was 102°F. We asked Mom to breastfeed while the baby cooled off and rehydrated. Ten or fifteen minutes later, we came back. Same baby, same room, but now he was calmly nursing, clothes dry, much more relaxed. We checked his temperature again: 99°F. Without any medicine, that fever dropped just by letting his body release the heat and by giving him fluids.

That visit became a turning point for the family. They could see with their own eyes that watching the child and creating the right conditions mattered more than chasing the highest number.

2. Safe Strategies for Fevers 102°+

When the fever is high enough to make your child miserable, typically above 102°F or when your child cannot settle for 30 minutes, my goal is comfort, not a perfectly "normal" temperature. We want to bring the fever down just enough so your child can rest and drink.

The "Slow Cool" Method

If your child feels like they are burning up, your instinct might be to put them in a cold bath. **Please do not do this.**

Cold water can shock the body and cause shivering. Shivering makes muscles work, which actually creates more heat and can raise the body temperature too much.

A better approach is a tepid bath. The water should feel slightly warm on the inside of your wrist—lukewarm, not hot and not cold. Gently sponge the water over their back and chest. As the water evaporates, it cools the skin naturally without triggering the shiver reflex.

Dressing for Success

Some people suggest bundling a child with a fever in heavy clothes or blankets to "sweat it out." This can be unsafe because it traps heat and may raise the body temperature too much.

Instead, dress your child in light cotton layers or just a diaper/underwear. If they have chills, add a light sheet or thin blanket, but keep the heavy comforter off until the fever breaks. Think "light and breathable," not "bundled and sweating."

When I think back to that bundled baby, I remember how shocked the parents were when I said, "Actually, less is more here." For them, unwrapping a hot child felt wrong, almost like bad parenting. Once they saw the temperature fall and their baby relax, the idea that heat needs a way out finally clicked. From then on, their first question at home became, "Is he overdressed?" instead of "How high is the number?"

The Medication Strategy (Integrative Approach)

Acetaminophen (Tylenol) and ibuprofen (Motrin/Advil) are tools you use when you need them, not daily vitamins. Be sure to follow dosing guidelines to avoid overlap. Acetaminophen can be given every 4–6 hours as needed, and ibuprofen can be given every 6-8 hours as needed. Always read and follow the package instructions or consult your provider.

When to use them: If the fever is keeping your child from drinking or sleeping. Sleep and hydration are more important than letting the fever run completely unchecked.

When you can wait: If your child's temperature is around 102°F and is playing quietly or sleeping peacefully, it is often safe to let the fever run its course.

Important safety note: Never give aspirin to children or teenagers. Aspirin is associated with Reye's Syndrome, a rare but serious condition that can affect the liver and brain.

3. Holistic Remedies: The Natural Toolkit

If you want to support the body without immediately suppressing the fever with medication, these natural methods are reasonable first steps. They can be used on their own or alongside conventional treatment.

Homeopathy: The "ABC" Trio

Homeopathic remedies are usually gentle and are often used alongside conventional medicine. Talk with your child's provider if you're unsure what's right for your family. These are options, not requirements; your comfort level matters.

- *Aconite (Aconitum napellus)*: Best when the fever comes on suddenly, often after exposure to cold, dry wind. The child may look anxious, restless, or fearful.

- *Belladonna*: For the "red, hot, and steaming" fever. The face is flushed, the skin is very warm, and the child may be sensitive to light and noise or a bit delirious.

- *Ferrum phos*: For the early stages of a milder, slower-building fever, before symptoms are dramatic.

The "Wet Sock" Treatment

The "wet sock" treatment may sound strange, but it's a classic naturopathic remedy many families use for congestion and high heat.

- *Warm the feet:* Soak your child's feet in warm water for about 5 minutes.

- *Cold layer:* Soak a pair of thin cotton socks in ice-cold water. Wring them out very well, then put them on the warm feet.

- *Warm layer:* Immediately pull a pair of dry, thick wool socks over the cold, wet cotton socks.

- *Bedtime:* Tuck your child into bed as usual.

Why it helps: When the feet are cold, the body increases blood flow there to warm them up. This can move blood and congestion away from the head and chest, which may ease pressure and help control temperature. By morning, the socks are usually dry. If your child doesn't like this treatment, you can skip it. It's just an option.

4. Hydration Hacks

A fever causes the body to use up energy and fluids more quickly. Dehydration is often a bigger problem than the fever itself.

The 15-Minute Rule

Don't push a full glass of water all at once. That often triggers vomiting in a feverish stomach. Instead, offer 1-2 teaspoons of fluid every 15 minutes. Small, frequent sips are easier to keep down.

"Nature's IV"

"Nature's IV": coconut water is often a better choice than plain water during illness because it contains natural electrolytes like potassium. If your child refuses coconut water, try:

- Diluted apple juice
- Broth
- Ice pops or ice chips

"Eating water" counts too. Think: anything wet and kid-approved beats nothing.

Output Check

A simple way to track whether your child is getting enough fluid is to watch their output. Fewer wet diapers, very dark urine, or no urination for 6-8 hours (in an older child) are reasons to check in with your pediatric provider.

5. Putting it All Together at 2 a.m.

When you're exhausted, it helps to think in steps rather than memorizing every detail.

A simple order of operations might look like this:

- First, look at your child, not just the number. Are they responsive? Breathing comfortably? Able to sip fluids?
- Second, lighten the load: remove extra layers, consider a lukewarm sponge bath, and make the room comfortably cool.
- Third, offer fluids in tiny, frequent sips following the 15-minute rule.
- Fourth, use medicine (acetaminophen or ibuprofen) if, and only if, the fever is clearly keeping them from drinking or sleeping.
- Finally, trust the process while watching for red flags (trouble breathing, unusual sleepiness, signs of dehydration)—those are the times to call for help.

You don't have to do everything perfectly. A few calm, simple steps are enough to support the body's built-in healing work.

6. When to Seek Medical Attention (Red Flags)

Most childhood fevers are uncomfortable but not dangerous. There are certain times, though, when you need medical help right away.

Age-Based Urgency

- *0–3 months*: Any fever above 100.4°F (rectal) is an emergency. Do not wait it out. Go to the ER. Young infants do not yet have the immune reserves to safely "watch and wait."

- *3–36 months*: Call your pediatrician for advice if the fever is around or above 102.2°F, especially if you are seeing any other concerning symptoms.

Remember the kindergartner from Chapter 1 who had 17 viral illnesses in his first school year? Many of those started with fevers that looked scary but followed a typical pattern and resolved safely with home care and monitoring.

Symptom Red Flags (Any Age)

Seek urgent care or emergency care if you see:

- *Neck stiffness*: Your child cannot touch their chin to their chest, or cries in pain when you try to move their neck.

- *Petechiae*: A rash of tiny red or purple spots that do not fade (blanch) when you press on them with your finger or a clear glass.

- *Breathing trouble*: Fast, labored breathing, flaring nostrils, or the skin pulling in between or under the ribs (retractions).

- *Lethargy*: Your child is very hard to wake up, won't look at you, or isn't acting like themselves at all.

- *Duration:* If a fever lasts longer than 3–5 days, your child should be checked by a doctor.

When you're not sure, I would rather you call or come in and have it be "nothing" than stay home worried and alone. You never have to apologize for asking for help.

Quick Guide: What To Do When Your Child Has a Fever

How to Take Your Child's Temperature

Use a digital thermometer to check your child's temperature. If your child won't keep the thermometer under their tongue, place it in their armpit, under their clothes, with their arm held gently against their side.

In my practice, I teach parents what I taught the bundled baby's family: under-arm with a digital thermometer is your safest, most realistic option at home. Rectal readings can be accurate, but I don't recommend them unless you're trained. Ear and forehead readings seem convenient, but in babies and toddlers, they are often misleading, especially if the ear itself is hot from crying or the skin is flushed from pushing blood to the surface to cool off.

Parents are often surprised to learn that a hat alone can make a difference. Younger children can lose a lot of heat through their heads. Taking the hat off and using the armpit for temperature gives you a truer sense of what is going on at the core.

When to Call, When to Go In

Think of fever decisions in three levels: call your provider, go to the ER, or call 911.

Call Your Pediatric Provider if:

- Your child has had a fever for 3 days in a row, and you don't see an obvious cause (like an ear infection or the flu).
- Your child isn't playing, seems confused, or is having trouble walking normally.
- Your child refuses to eat or drink.
- Your child has had a fever, and you're worried, even if you're not sure why.

Go to the ER if:

- An infant under 1 month of age has a fever over about 100.7°F.
- An older child has a temperature over about 103.5°F, and it is not coming down at all with fever reducers.
- Your child seems severely dehydrated (very dry mouth, little or no urine, dark yellow urine, crying without tears, weak or dizzy, or a sunken soft spot in infants).
- Your child has a seizure.
- Your child has a fever over 105°F.

Call 911 if:

- Your child has a seizure that lasts 5 minutes or longer.
- Your child will not wake up.
- Your child is too weak to move or stand.

If you're ever unsure, trust your instincts. If something seems very wrong, it's always okay to get help right away.

USING FEVER REDUCERS SAFELY

Acetaminophen (Tylenol) and ibuprofen (Motrin/Advil) can be used to reduce a fever and help with comfort.

- For babies under 1 month of age, always contact your pediatric provider before giving any fever reducer.
- For older babies and children, follow the dosing chart from your pediatrician or the package, based on weight.

The goal is not to "chase" every degree, but to help your child feel well enough to drink, rest, and recover. Think "more comfortable," not "perfectly normal."

WHAT THIS LOOKS LIKE IN REAL LIFE

For babies like the bundled 8-month-old, our aftercare plan was simple: dress in a light onesie, avoid heavy blankets, breastfeed frequently to maintain hydration, check the under-arm temperature periodically, and call us if the temperature climbed back to 102°F and the baby looked worse. The fever never returned to that level once the heat could escape and fluids were going in.

For toddlers and preschoolers, the conversation sounds a little different. I often tell parents, "Toddlers are professional complainers." If a 3- or 4-year-old with a temperature of only 100°F is miserable, whiny, saying 'I don't feel good' and just wants to sleep on the couch, it is okay to give a dose of acetaminophen or ibuprofen for comfort. You are not ruining their immune response; you are helping them rest, drink, and conserve energy so their body can keep doing the hard work.

WHAT NOT TO DO

Avoid older home methods that can be harmful:

- Do not use ice packs or alcohol baths to bring down a fever. These are no longer recommended and can have adverse effects.

- Do not overdress your child or pile on heavy blankets. This can trap heat and raise their temperature.

Instead, keep them in light clothing, offer plenty of fluids, and use the "slow cool" and medication strategies from earlier in this chapter.

Watching for Dehydration

Keep an eye out for signs of dehydration, especially when your child has a fever:

- Dry mouth or lips
- Little or no urine, or very dark yellow urine
- Crying without tears
- Weakness or dizziness
- Sunken soft spot on the head (in infants)
- Sunken eyes or cheeks

If you notice these signs, increase their fluid intake and call your provider for guidance.

A Note on Essential Oils

Some families like to use essential oils as part of their home care. For children aged 2 and older, some parents gently rub diluted peppermint essential oil on the back or the bottoms of the feet. If you use oils:

- Always dilute them in a carrier oil (like coconut or olive oil).
- Never apply strong oils directly to a child's face or near their eyes or nose.
- Stop right away if your child seems irritated by the scent or develops redness.

Always ask your child's provider if you're unsure about using essential oils in your home. If your pediatrician disagrees with using essential oils, follow their guidance for your child.

School and Activity

Children with fevers should stay home from school or daycare and rest. They should drink plenty of fluids and avoid heavy activity until they are better.

If you don't yet know what is causing the fever, monitor your child closely for changes in their behavior, breathing, and hydration, not just the thermometer reading.

Once the fever breaks, the cough usually begins. In the next chapter, we'll tackle the sounds that keep the whole house awake: persistent coughs and sore throats, and how to tell when they are just annoying and when they need more attention. You'll learn which coughs can wait for morning and which ones need a call right away.

Most childhood fevers are uncomfortable, but with the right information, they don't have to feel terrifying. When you understand that fever is often the body's way of fighting for your child, not against them, it becomes easier to watch the number on the thermometer without panicking at every climb. You now know when to comfort and hydrate at home, when to pick up the phone, and when a fever truly needs urgent care.

When you find yourself awake at 2 a.m. with a hot little body on your chest, you can come back to a few simple questions: How does my child look? Are they drinking at least a little? Are they breathing comfortably? Is this following a typical pattern, or is something different this time? Those questions will serve you better than staring at a single number on a screen.

If the answers worry you, call. If the answers reassure you, lean on the tools you now have—light layers, slow cooling, fluids, and medicine when your child truly needs comfort—and let their immune system do its work. You are not expected to be a walking textbook. You are expected to notice, to care, and to ask for help when your gut says something is off.

In the next chapter, we'll follow the story where fever often leaves off. Once the temperature starts to settle, the cough usually ramps up: the barking fits at 2 a.m., the sore throats that make every swallow hurt, and the ear pains that show up just as everyone tries to sleep. We'll walk through which coughs can safely wait for morning, which sore throats and earaches need to be seen, and how to use simple tools at home to ease symptoms without shutting down the body's natural cleanup process.

Fever is the heat of the battle. Coughs, sore throats, and ear infections are often the cleanup crew. By the time you turn the page, you'll be ready for both.

REFERENCES

Arnon, S. S., Schechter, R., Inglesby, T. V., Henderson, D. A., Bartlett, J. G., Ascher, M. S., Eitzen, E., Fine, A. D., Hauer, J., Layton, M., Lillibridge, S., Osterholm, M. T., O'Toole, T., Parker, G., Perl, T. M., Russell, P. K., Swerdlow, D. L., & Tonat, K. (2001). Botulinum toxin as a biological weapon: Medical and public health management. JAMA, 285(8), 1059–1070. *https://doi.org/10.1001/jama.285.8.1059*

Chang, A. B., Glomb, W. B. (2001). A review of cough in children. The Journal of Asthma, 38(4), 299–309. *https://doi.org/10.1081/JAS-100103781*

Chang, A. B., Oppenheimer, J. J., Irwin, R. S., & CHEST Expert Cough Panel. (2020). Managing chronic cough as a symptom in children and management algorithms: CHEST guideline and expert panel report. Chest, 158(1), 303–329. *https://doi.org/10.1016/j.chest.2020.01.042*

Cohen, H. A., Rozen, J., Kristal, H., Laks, Y., Berkovitch, M., Uziel, Y., Kozer, E., Pomeranz, A., & Efrat, H. (2012). Effect of honey on nocturnal cough and sleep quality: A double-blind, randomized, placebo-controlled study. Pediatrics, 130(3), 465–471. *https://doi.org/10.1542/peds.2011-3075*

Hao, Q., Dong, B. R., & Wu, T. (2015). Probiotics for preventing acute upper respiratory tract infections. Cochrane Database of Systematic Reviews, 2015(2), CD006895. *https://doi.org/10.1002/14651858.CD006895.pub3*

Lieberthal, A. S., Carroll, A. E., Chonmaitree, T., Ganiats, T. G., Hoberman, A., Jackson, M. A., Joffe, M. D., Miller, D. T., Rosenfeld, R. M., Sevilla, X. D., Schwartz, R. H., Thomas, P. A., & Tunkel, D. E. (2013). The diagnosis and management of acute otitis media. Pediatrics, 131(3), e964–e999. *https://doi.org/10.1542/peds.2012-3488*

Paul, I. M., Beiler, J., McMonagle, A., Shaffer, M. L., Duda, L., & Berlin, C. M., Jr. (2007). Effect of honey, dextromethorphan, and no treatment on nocturnal cough and sleep quality for coughing children and their parents. Archives of Pediatrics & Adolescent Medicine, 161(12), 1140–1146. *https://doi.org/10.1001/archpedi.161.12.1140*

Sarrell, E. M., Mandelberg, A., & Cohen, H. A. (2001). Efficacy of naturopathic extracts in the management of ear pain associated with acute otitis media. Archives of Pediatrics & Adolescent Medicine, 155(7), 796–799. *https://doi.org/10.1001/archpedi.155.7.796*

Szajewska, H., Hojsak, I., Kolacek, S., Orel, R., Shomarova, D., Tindberg, Y., Weizman, Z., & Vandenplas, Y. (2016). Probiotics for the prevention of antibiotic-associated diarrhea in children. Journal of Pediatric Gastroenterology and Nutrition, 62(3), 495–506. *https://doi.org/10.1097/MPG.0000000000001012*

Thompson, M., Vodicka, T. A., Blair, P. S., Buckley, D. I., Heneghan, C., & Hay, A. D. (2013). Duration of symptoms of respiratory tract infections in children: Systematic review. BMJ, 347, f7027. *https://doi.org/10.1136/bmj.f7027*

CHAPTER 3

PERSISTENT COUGH, SORE THROAT & EAR INFECTIONS

There is no sound more helpless for a parent than the dry, hacking bark of a cough echoing through the house at 2 a.m. It disrupts sleep for everyone, and the sheer force of it can be frightening to witness in a young child.

Our instinct is to stop the cough immediately. We want to shut it down so they (and we) can finally sleep. But it helps to remember the biological purpose behind it: the cough is the broom.

In the last chapter, we talked about how fever is often the body's way of fighting for your child, not against them. Once that fever starts to settle, the noisy, lingering cough you hear at 2 a.m. is usually the next stage of that same healing process, helping clear out everything the immune system has been working on.

Coughing is the body's main way of clearing mucus, dead cells, and trapped germs out of the lungs. When we completely shut down the cough reflex, all that gunk can sit in the airways longer, which may increase the risk of pneumonia or other infections. However, it is essential to note that in rare situations—such as when dealing with an immunocompromised child or a child with chronic lung disease—suppressing a cough may be appropriate and necessary under medical guidance. These exceptions should be carefully considered to prevent confusion regarding general advice.

Since COVID, I have seen parents become more anxious about every cough. We are noticing patterns more, not because coughs are new or worse, but because families are coming in sooner and more often to ask, "Is this still normal?" This chapter aims to answer that question with practical advice, showing how to ease coughs, sore throats, and ear pain without stopping the body's natural cleaning process, and how to know when to call the doctor or ask about antibiotics.

1. Natural Relief for Coughs and Sore Throats

Before reaching for over-the-counter cough syrups, many of which are not recommended for younger children due to side effects and limited benefit, it can be helpful to start with gentle, age-appropriate home care. These strategies are meant to help you feel confident that you are soothing your child in safe and effective ways.

The Golden Spoon: Honey

For older children, honey can be very helpful at night. Studies show it can be as effective as, or even better than, common cough suppressants for calming nighttime coughs. Honey coats the throat, soothes irritated nerves, and has mild antimicrobial effects.

How to use. Give your child one-half to one teaspoon of dark honey (Buckwheat or Manuka are especially strong, but any dark honey works) about 30 minutes before bed or during a coughing fit. Let them slowly lick it from the spoon or mix it into warm water or herbal tea.

Critical safety. Never give honey to a child under 12 months old due to the risk of infant botulism. Babies' digestive systems are not mature enough to safely handle the spores naturally present in honey.

Steam and Humidity

The "steam tent:" If your child has a "barky," seal-like cough (often heard with croup) or a dry, tickly cough, taking them into a steamy bathroom can work wonders. Turn on the hot shower, close the door, and sit on the toilet or floor with your child for 10–15 minutes. The warm, moist air helps relax the vocal cords and airways, easing the intensity of the cough.

Cool mist at night: Use a cool-mist humidifier in your child's bedroom while they sleep. Dry air can make a sore throat feel worse, while humidity soothes it. Be sure to clean the humidifier regularly as the manufacturer recommends, so you do not spread mold or bacteria. Maintain room humidity levels between 50 to 75% for best results.

The Saltwater Gargle

For children old enough to understand "swish and spit" (usually around age four and up), a warm saltwater gargle is one of the oldest and most reliable tricks for sore throats.

The mix: Dissolve one-half teaspoon of salt in 8 ounces of warm water.

Why it helps: Salt pulls water out of swollen throat tissues, which can reduce pain. Gargling also helps rinse away mucus and virus particles from the back of the throat. Many kids like that they can do something themselves to help their throat feel better.

What I See With Persistent Coughs

Since COVID, I see far more families coming in for "this cough just won't go away." Sometimes the cough really is lasting longer; often it has always lasted that long, but no one came in at week three before the pandemic. One of the most common patterns I see is simple post-nasal drip.

Inside the nose are two structures called turbinates. When a child is sick or exposed to things like pollution or smoke, the turbinates swell. Instead of mucus draining out the front, it runs down the back of the throat, especially when lying down. This drip can tickle the throat and cause a cough. Kids may wake up coughing, gagging, or sounding like they are choking, which can look dramatic, but the real problem is often in the nose, not the lungs.

In these cases, focus on thinning and moving the mucus. Use saline sprays or rinses, xylitol nasal sprays, steam, and make sure your child stays well hydrated. Research shows that saltwater or xylitol rinses help clear the turbinates and reduce post-nasal drip. When we clean the upper airway, the cough often gets better in a few days without strong medications.

QUICK GUIDE: WHEN TO SEEK CARE FOR A CHILD'S COUGH

Coughs are very common in children and are usually caused by viral illnesses. Most get better on their own with time and simple care at home. This chapter is meant to help you decide when to call your child's doctor and when symptoms are serious enough to need emergency care. Remember the kindergartner in Chapter 1 who had 17 viral illnesses in his first school year: many of them showed up as a runny nose and a lingering cough that resolved with time, fluids, and the home tools you will find in this chapter.

Call the Office or Schedule a Visit if Your Child Has:

- A cough lasting more than 4 weeks (chronic cough)
- A cough that is not improving or is getting worse after 10–14 days
- A cough with fever lasting more than 3 days or with fever that keeps coming back
- A nighttime cough that wakes your child regularly
- A cough with wheezing, chest tightness, or shortness of breath during activity
- A cough associated with vomiting, poor appetite, or weight loss
- A cough that begins after a choking episode

- A history of asthma, allergies, or recurrent pneumonia, and now has a new or persistent cough
- A cough that is interfering with sleep, school, or daily activities

Go to the Emergency Room or Call 911 if Your Child Has:

- Trouble breathing, fast breathing, or working hard to breathe (ribs pulling in, belly breathing, flaring nostrils)
- A blue or gray color to the lips, face, or fingernails
- Stridor (a high-pitched noise when breathing in) or severe wheezing
- Sudden onset of coughing or breathing trouble, especially if choking is suspected
- Coughing up blood
- Lethargy, confusion, or difficulty waking up
- An infant under 3 months old with a cough and any fever
- A cough with severe chest pain or fainting

Helpful Reminders

- Honey may be used for cough only in children over 1 year of age. Remember, one candle on the cake, then honey's okay. This rhythmic reminder helps avoid mistakes when you're tired.
- Avoid smoke and vaping exposure around your child
- Over-the-counter cough and cold medicines are not recommended for young children.

If you are unsure or concerned, trust your instincts and seek care. I would always rather have you call with a question than sit at home, worried and alone.

2. Home Remedies That Work for Kids

Chest Rubs (The Aromatic Approach)

Many traditional vapor rubs contain camphor or very strong menthol, which can be too intense for young airways and may even trigger breathing spasms in babies.

The gentler option: Choose a child-safe chest rub or make your own using milder essential oils such as *eucalyptus radiata* (a gentler species than *eucalyptus globulus*), pine, or fir, all well diluted in a carrier oil like coconut or olive oil.

How to apply:

- For older children, rub a small amount on their chest and upper back to create a gentle feeling of warmth and comfort.

- For babies or kids with sensitive skin, apply the rub to the soles of the feet and cover with socks. The oils are still absorbed without irritating the eyes or nose.

Always keep essential oils out of reach, never let a child ingest them, and check with your child's provider if you are unsure which products are safe for their age.

The "Propped Up" Sleep

Gravity can make things worse when your child is congested. Lying flat lets mucus collect in the back of the throat, which can cause gagging or coughing.

Tip: Slightly raise the head of the mattress by placing a rolled towel or firm pillow under the top of it—not under your child's head, as that can be unsafe for babies and cause neck strain in older kids. A gentle angle of fifteen to thirty degrees helps the sinuses drain while they sleep.

Warm Fluids vs. Cold Popsicles

Warm options: Kid-safe herbal teas such as chamomile or "throat" blends can relax throat muscles, thin mucus, and make coughs more productive and less painful. Add a little honey for children over one year of age if your provider agrees.

Cold options: If the throat is very raw, red, and swollen (as in strep throat or Hand, Foot, and Mouth disease), a cold treat may feel better than a warm compress. Ice pops made from real fruit juice or cooled herbal tea act like tiny numbing sticks for the back of the throat and also boost fluid intake.

Follow your child's lead, as some kids crave warm, while others prefer icy. Both can be helpful tools.

A Story About Finding the Root Cause

One of the more memorable "mystery cough" cases in my practice was a school-age boy with a cough that would not quit. It started near the end of the school year and lingered straight into summer. His mom noticed something curious: the cough was much worse when he spent time indoors and almost disappeared on beach days. At the ocean, his cough went down to nearly zero.

When I examined him, his lungs sounded clear. What I consistently saw was swollen nasal turbinates and post-nasal drip, not pneumonia, not asthma, just persistent upper airway irritation. That told me something in his everyday environment was constantly triggering mucus production.

We went through a long list together: pets, plants, laundry detergents, scented cleaners, plug-in air fresheners. The only thing that stood out was a pet turtle tank in his bedroom. Turtles can harbor bacteria such as *E. coli* and *Pseudomonas*, and in a closed room can become a constant, low-level irritant. We moved the turtle out of his room. Within weeks, his cough calmed down. It never progressed to an ear infection or a sore throat, because we finally removed the trigger.

I share that story not because every persistent cough is a turtle problem, but to show how often the "mystery" is in the air your child breathes. Sometimes the most potent treatment is changing what they are breathing in every night.

Air Quality, Humidity, and Essential Oils

I care a lot about air quality at home and at work. Parents often worry about mold, but there are many simple things you can do before considering a mold inspection. The easiest is to open a window. In some European countries, people open their windows every day, even in cold weather, to let in fresh air. You can try this at home too.

At home, I use HEPA air purifiers in most major rooms and monitor humidity. When humidity drops below about thirty percent, the air becomes bone dry. You feel it in your nose and on your skin. Dry mucous membranes crack, cannot trap germs as well, and make coughs more painful. A cool-mist humidifier during dry seasons, especially at night, can help keep humidity in a more comfortable range and support the throat and nose in recovering.

For essential oils to help with coughs and congestion, choose reputable brands that test their products. Off-brand oils can vary in quality, and with kids, you want to avoid surprises. Blends with lemon, eucalyptus, and lavender in a diffuser can help thin mucus and make breathing easier. Most major brands have a 'breathe' or 'respiratory' blend for this. Always use a diffuser in a well-ventilated room, and do not put strong oils directly on your child's skin or near their face unless you know how to dilute them safely.

3. EAR INFECTIONS: DETECTION, CARE, AND "WATCHFUL WAITING."

Ear infections (acute otitis media) are one of the most common reasons children are prescribed antibiotics. The important message for parents is this: not every earache automatically needs antibiotics, and you do not have to make that call alone.

Why It Happens

Children's Eustachian tubes, the tiny "drain pipes" of the ear, are shorter and more horizontal than those of adults. When a child has a cold or allergies, fluid can get trapped in the middle ear like water in a clogged sink. If that fluid sits too long, bacteria can grow and cause an infection.

The upper airway is a single connected pathway: the ears, nose, throat, and sinuses. When a parent brings in a child with a two-week cough and a sore throat, and now they are tugging at their ear, I know the same inflammatory process is likely affecting all of those areas. Mucus that starts in the nose can flow back up the Eustachian tube and into the middle ear. That is often how a simple cold turns into an ear infection over seven to ten days.

Early Detection

Because little ones can't always say, "My ear hurts," you'll want to watch for signs such as:

- Tugging or pulling at the ears
- Increased fussiness or crying, especially when lying flat (pressure in the ear rises in that position)
- Trouble sleeping or sudden waking with crying
- Older kids complaining of ear fullness, popping, or pain
- Fluid draining from the ear (this may mean the eardrum has perforated—see a doctor immediately)

If you see these signs, check in with your child's healthcare provider for an exam and advice.

In this situation, I cannot diagnose over text or video. I need to look in your child's ears and throat, and sometimes swab the throat, to see if it is a lingering virus, a new bacterial infection like strep, or both. If your child has a persistent cough, sore throat, and is pulling at their ears, bring them in for a visit.

The Garlic & Mullein Oil Trick

In many holistic pediatric practices, garlic and mullein oil ear drops are used as a gentle support when appropriate. Garlic has antimicrobial properties; mullein flowers are known for their soothing, pain-relieving effects.

How to use: Warm the bottle in your hands (never in the microwave) until it is just slightly warm. Have your child lie on their side with the sore ear facing up. Place two to three drops in the affected ear, then keep them in that position for about five minutes so the oil can coat the canal.

Important safety: Do not use ear drops if there is any discharge from the ear, if you think the eardrum is perforated, or if your child has ear tubes. In these cases, your child needs a medical evaluation instead of home ear drops. Always follow your provider's advice.

Lymphatic Massage

You can gently encourage fluid to drain away from the ears by helping the lymphatic system along.

With clean hands, use your fingertips to gently massage just behind your child's earlobe in small circles, then stroke downward along the big neck muscle (the sternocleidomastoid) toward the collarbone. Use light pressure and a slow, soothing motion. A minute or two on each side, a few times a day, can feel calming and may support drainage.

4. The Strategy: "Watchful Waiting" vs. Antibiotics

For many otherwise healthy children, especially those over age two with mild symptoms, pediatric guidelines support a "watchful waiting" period of forty-eight to seventy-two hours before starting antibiotics for certain ear infections. Your child's provider will help determine whether this is appropriate in your situation.

Why Wait?

- Many ear infections are viral, and antibiotics do not treat viruses.
- Even some bacterial ear infections will resolve on their own as congestion clears and fluid drains.
- Avoiding antibiotics when they are not needed protects your child's gut microbiome and helps prevent antibiotic resistance over time.

During the wait, your job is to keep your child as comfortable as possible and watch for improvement or worsening. This may include:

- Pain relievers such as acetaminophen or ibuprofen, if recommended by your provider
- Warm compresses over the ear
- Garlic–mullein oil drops when appropriate and approved
- Extra fluids, rest, and cuddles

When to Treat with Antibiotics

Your child's healthcare provider may recommend starting antibiotics right away, or after a brief period of watchful waiting, if any of the following are present:

- Pain or fever worsens or does not improve after forty-eight to seventy-two hours
- Your child is under 6 months old with a suspected ear infection

- Your child appears very unwell or "toxic" (very lethargic, high persistent fever, inconsolable pain)

- Both ears are infected, especially in younger children

- There are repeated ear infections or underlying medical conditions that make complications more likely

When antibiotics are needed, they can be truly lifesaving. The goal is not to avoid them at all costs, but to use them wisely, at the right time, for the right child.

5. Supporting Recovery: The Art of Convalescence

In our fast-paced world, it is tempting to send kids back to school, daycare, or sports the moment the fever breaks and they seem a little better. Unfortunately, this can set them up for a setback.

Convalescence is the quiet recovery phase. A child getting over a respiratory virus still has depleted energy reserves and an immune system that is finishing the job behind the scenes. Sending them back to busy environments too soon can make them more vulnerable to a secondary infection (like bacterial pneumonia) or a relapse of their original illness.

A helpful rule of thumb: Once your child is acting like themselves again, give them one extra "boring day" at home, no big outings, no intense practices, before returning to normal activities. Think of it as a buffer that lets their body fully catch up.

Post-Antibiotic Care

If antibiotics were necessary (and sometimes they absolutely are), healing continues even after the last dose. Antibiotics are like a controlled forest fire: they burn down harmful bacteria, but they also affect many of the helpful ones living in your child's gut.

To support rebuilding:

- Probiotics: Ask your child's provider about a high-quality probiotic with strains such as *Lactobacillus rhamnosus* or *Saccharomyces boulardii* that are appropriate for your child's age.
- Timing: Give the probiotic at least two hours away from the antibiotic dose (for example, antibiotic at 8:00 AM, probiotic at 10:00 AM). If you give them together, the antibiotic can kill the probiotic before it has a chance to help.
- Duration: Continue the probiotic for about two weeks after the antibiotic course is finished, unless your child's provider gives different instructions.

You can also focus on nourishing foods, such as yogurt with live cultures (for children who tolerate dairy), fruits, vegetables, and plenty of fluids, to gently support the body's healing process.

Coughs, sore throats, and ear infections are some of the most common reasons children need comfort in the middle of the night. They can seem dramatic and look scary, but now you have a better idea of what is normal, what you can safely manage at home, and when to seek medical care. With simple tools like honey, steam, positioning, gentle ear care, and a plan for watchful waiting or antibiotics, you can feel more prepared and less helpless.

When your child is coughing in the middle of the night, pulling at their ear, or whispering that their throat hurts, you do not have to wonder unthinkingly, "Is this okay?" You know how to listen for their breathing, look at their energy, and decide whether tonight calls for home care, a call to the office, or a visit in person. You also know that sometimes the answer is not another medicine at all, but opening a window, running a humidifier, or moving the turtle tank out of the bedroom.

In the next chapter, we zoom out from these middle-of-the-night emergencies and ask a different question: how do we give your child fewer of them in the first place? We will look at how everyday food choices, hydration, the "no-naked-carb" rule, the rainbow on the plate, and a few well-chosen supplements can quietly train the immune system long before the first cough starts.

If this chapter has been about putting out fires safely, Chapter four is about building a home that is harder to set on fire at all.

REFERENCES

Arnon, S. S., Schechter, R., Inglesby, T. V., Henderson, D. A., Bartlett, J. G., Ascher, M. S., Eitzen, E., Fine, A. D., Hauer, J., Layton, M., Lillibridge, S., Osterholm, M. T., O'Toole, T., Parker, G., Perl, T. M., Russell, P. K., Swerdlow, D. L., & Tonat, K. (2001). Botulinum toxin as a biological weapon: Medical and public health management. JAMA, 285(8), 1059–1070. *https://doi.org/10.1001/jama.285.8.1059*

Chang, A. B., Glomb, W. B. (2001). A review of cough in children. The Journal of Asthma, 38(4), 299–309. *https://doi.org/10.1081/JAS-100103781*

Chang, A. B., Oppenheimer, J. J., Irwin, R. S., & CHEST Expert Cough Panel. (2020). Managing chronic cough as a symptom in children and management algorithms: CHEST guideline and expert panel report. Chest, 158(1), 303–329. *https://doi.org/10.1016/j.chest.2020.01.042*

Cohen, H. A., Rozen, J., Kristal, H., Laks, Y., Berkovitch, M., Uziel, Y., Kozer, E., Pomeranz, A., & Efrat, H. (2012). Effect of honey on nocturnal cough and sleep quality: A double-blind, randomized, placebo-controlled study. Pediatrics, 130(3), 465–471. *https://doi.org/10.1542/peds.2011-3075*

Hao, Q., Dong, B. R., & Wu, T. (2015). Probiotics for preventing acute upper respiratory tract infections. Cochrane Database of Systematic Reviews, 2015(2), CD006895. *https://doi.org/10.1002/14651858.CD006895.pub3*

Lieberthal, A. S., Carroll, A. E., Chonmaitree, T., Ganiats, T. G., Hoberman, A., Jackson, M. A., Joffe, M. D., Miller, D. T., Rosenfeld, R. M., Sevilla, X. D., Schwartz, R. H., Thomas, P. A., & Tunkel, D. E. (2013). The diagnosis and management of acute otitis media. Pediatrics, 131(3), e964–e999. *https://doi.org/10.1542/peds.2012-3488*

Paul, I. M., Beiler, J., McMonagle, A., Shaffer, M. L., Duda, L., & Berlin, C. M., Jr. (2007). Effect of honey, dextromethorphan, and no treatment on nocturnal cough and sleep quality for coughing children and their parents. Archives of Pediatrics & Adolescent Medicine, 161(12), 1140–1146. *https://doi.org/10.1001/archpedi.161.12.1140*

Sarrell, E. M., Mandelberg, A., & Cohen, H. A. (2001). Efficacy of naturopathic extracts in the management of ear pain associated with acute otitis media. Archives of Pediatrics & Adolescent Medicine, 155(7), 796–799. *https://doi.org/10.1001/archpedi.155.7.796*

Szajewska, H., Hojsak, I., Kolacek, S., Orel, R., Shomarova, D., Tindberg, Y., Weizman, Z., & Vandenplas, Y. (2016). Probiotics for the prevention of antibiotic-associated diarrhea in children. Journal of Pediatric Gastroenterology and Nutrition, 62(3), 495–506. *https://doi.org/10.1097/MPG.0000000000001012*

Thompson, M., Vodicka, T. A., Blair, P. S., Buckley, D. I., Heneghan, C., & Hay, A. D. (2013). Duration of symptoms of respiratory tract infections in children: Systematic review. BMJ, 347, f7027. *https://doi.org/10.1136/bmj.f7027*

CHAPTER 4

NUTRITION & IMMUNE-BOOSTING TIPS

Consistent mealtime habits can lead to fewer sick days for your child. Real immunity, which keeps your child healthier, is crafted long before the first sneeze—at the dinner table, in the lunchbox, and over breakfast. Think of your child's immune system as an army and food as its supply line. Just like an army needs fuel and supplies to work well, your child's body needs the right foods to stay strong. This chapter gives you simple, practical ways to help protect your child before and during cold and flu season.

One early experience changed how I talk about nutrition with families. Two siblings, about six and eight years old, came in looking very thin. Their weights were far below the growth chart, and their bones were visible under their skin. When I spoke with their mother, she told me she had a severe eating disorder and was afraid of passing it on to her children. To protect them, she had limited their diet so much that, for a long time, they ate only apples and drank water. They were malnourished, not because she didn't care, but because she was scared. We worked together with her, their dad, and a nutritionist to slowly add more foods back into their diet. Once their meals were balanced again, the kids did very well. That family showed me how important it is to explain nutrition in simple, clear terms that respect both science and the real worries parents have.

That's what this chapter aims to do: give you clear, realistic advice on what to put on your child's plate—from colorful foods to supplements and snacks—that helps their immune system every day.

1. THE "RAINBOW" RULE: IMMUNE-SUPPORTING FOODS

The immune system is hungry for nutrients. It needs a constant supply of micronutrients to produce white blood cells, antibodies, and anti-inflammatory compounds. Aim for a rainbow on your child's plate, as colorful foods naturally cover a wide range of nutrients.

Orange & Yellow (The Barrier Builders)

Foods: Sweet potatoes, carrots, oranges, pumpkin, and yellow bell peppers.

Why they matter: These foods are rich in beta-carotene (which the body converts to Vitamin A) and Vitamin C. Vitamin A is crucial for keeping your child's skin and nasal linings strong, acting as a barrier against infection. When Vitamin A levels are low, these protective linings can become thin and dry, making it easier for viruses to enter the body.

Kid hack: Make "hidden veggie" mac and cheese by blending boiled carrots or butternut squash into the cheese sauce. You add a big dose of Vitamin A without a fight.

Deep Greens (The Cell Repairers)

Foods: Spinach, broccoli, kale.

Why they matter: These greens are packed with magnesium, folate, and Vitamin K. They support DNA repair, help regulate inflammation, and keep the immune system from getting stuck in a constant "on" position.

Kid hack: If your child refuses salad, don't force it. Blend a handful of spinach into a berry smoothie. The blueberries hide the green color, and the taste disappears.

Red & Blue (The Firefighters)

Foods: Berries (strawberries, blueberries), red grapes, tomatoes, cherries.

Why they matter: Their bright colors signal flavonoids and antioxidants. When the immune system fights a virus, it creates oxidative stress (like exhaust fumes from an engine). Antioxidants help clean up those fumes so the immune system can keep running without burning out.

Kid hack: Freeze-dried strawberries or blueberries are crunchy like chips but retain most of their nutrients. They make an easy, shelf-stable snack.

White & Brown (The Gut Feeders)

Foods: Onions, garlic, oats, chickpeas, mushrooms.

Why they matter: These contain prebiotics, food for the good bacteria in your child's gut, and minerals like zinc. Garlic is naturally antimicrobial. Since about 70% of the immune system lives in the gut, feeding those good bacteria is like reinforcing the walls of the castle from the inside.

Kid hack: Make "superhero garlic bread" by mixing a little minced garlic into butter or olive oil and spreading it on whole-grain toast. Or, stir cooked onions and mushrooms into spaghetti sauce or taco meat, where they blend in and mostly disappear.

From First Bites to Picky Phases

From the first solids at around 6 months, I encourage families to think "from the ground up": foods that grow out of the ground, plus simple, lean proteins. That means fruits, vegetables, beans, and lean proteins like shredded chicken and flaky fish rather than processed, boxed foods. Babies are often more adventurous than we expect. They will usually try almost anything you offer in that first year; the real picky phase tends to show up between ages three and five. If you lay a foundation of whole foods early, they have a much better chance of returning to those foods after the picky years pass.

2. Core Supplements: Your "Winter Insurance Policy."

Ideally, your child would get everything they need from food. Modern soil depletion, indoor lifestyles, picky eating, and busy schedules mean there can be gaps. Think of these supplements not as replacements for good food, but as an insurance policy during cold and flu season.

For a more budget-friendly approach, consider affordable options like canned salmon for its rich omega-3 content or spend time outdoors on sunny days to naturally boost Vitamin D levels.

Always talk with your pediatric provider before starting new supplements, especially if your child has medical conditions, allergies, or takes regular medications.

Vitamin D3 + K2 (The Foundation)

Most children are low in Vitamin D, especially in winter when sunlight is weak, and kids are indoors. Vitamin D behaves more like a hormone than a vitamin; it helps activate T-cells, the "soldiers" that recognize and attack infected cells. Liquid drops are easiest and most flexible. Look for D3 paired with K2, which helps guide calcium into bones instead of soft tissues.

In my practice, I recommend vitamin D very early. For infants, that can mean 400 IU of D3 daily directly for the baby, or 4,000–5,000 IU for a breastfeeding parent, so enough D comes through the milk. As kids grow and start eating regular foods, keeping vitamin D on board continues to support immune function and bone health at the same time.

Zinc (The Gatekeeper)

Zinc is crucial for the thymus gland, where immune cells mature. It also supports the integrity of the respiratory tract lining, the tissue first exposed to airborne viruses.

How to use it: Zinc lozenges or liquid can be helpful at the very first signs of illness (scratchy throat, first sniffles). Early use may shorten the course or lessen severity.

Caution: Always give zinc with food to avoid nausea, and avoid long-term high dosing without medical guidance.

Probiotics (The Headquarters)

Because much of the immune system sits in the gut, a healthy microbiome is central to immune resilience.

Strains to consider: Look for kid-friendly products that include strains such as *Lactobacillus rhamnosus* GG and *Bifidobacterium* species, both of which have research support for gut and immune health.

When to use: Daily during winter, and especially after a course of antibiotics to help rebuild healthy gut flora.

Elderberry (The Viral Blocker)

Black elderberry (*Sambucus nigra*) has been studied for its ability to interfere with viral replication. It doesn't prevent exposure, but it may help reduce how quickly a virus multiplies.

Best timing: Use at the very first sign of illness, when your child seems "off," has a mild sore throat, or on the first day of a cold. Starting it late in the illness is less effective.

Forms: Syrups and gummies are common and generally well-accepted by kids.

3. Hydration: The Forgotten Nutrient

When your child is well-hydrated, their mucus stays thin and can help trap and remove germs. If they are dehydrated, their mucus gets thick and sticky, which can let germs grow instead of blocking them. Staying hydrated is more important than many people think. Plain, filtered water should be your child's main drink. Milk and foods with lots of water can help, but sugary drinks can actually harm immune health.

Daily Fluid Targets by Age (Approximate)

These are general guidelines; needs vary with activity and climate.

Age Group	Recommended Daily Fluid Intake (Total)
Infants (0–6 months)	Breast milk or formula provides all the needed fluids.
Toddlers (1–3 years)	About 4 cups (32 oz) of fluids total.
School Age (4–8 years)	About 5 cups (40 oz) of fluids total.
Older Children (9–13)	Girls: ~7 cups (56 oz). Boys: ~8 cups (64 oz).

Total fluids include water, milk, and water-rich foods, but the bulk should be plain water.

Hydration Hacks

- Keep water bottles visible: in the car, by the bed, on the homework table, in the backpack.
- Offer water with every snack and meal.

- Use herbal teas (chamomile, hibiscus, peppermint for older kids) as cozy, caffeine-free options.
- Make simple ice pops with diluted juice or herbal tea for kids who resist drinking.

QUICK GUIDE: DAILY NUTRITION CHECKLIST FOR IMMUNE SUPPORT

You don't have to be perfect. Try to meet most of these goals on most days.

Food & Color

- Add at least one orange/yellow food
- Include at least one deep green food (even if blended)
- Serve at least one red or blue fruit or vegetable
- Incorporate at least one white/brown "gut feeder" (onion, garlic, oats, beans, mushrooms)
- Ensure protein at each meal
- Include a source of healthy fat (nuts, seeds, avocado, olive oil, fatty fish)

Fluids

- Provide age-appropriate total fluids, with water as the main drink
- Minimize sugary beverages

Optional Immune Supports (If approved by your child's provider)

- Administer daily Vitamin D3 (especially in winter)

- Give probiotic most days
- Use zinc and elderberry at the first sign of illness

4. Quick Nutrition Strategies for Busy Parents

You don't need fancy recipes to help your child's immunity. Simple daily habits make a big difference.

The "Power Sprinkle"

Mix hemp seeds, chia seeds, and ground flax in a small jar and keep it on the counter. Sprinkle it on oatmeal, yogurt, peanut butter toast, smoothies, or cottage cheese. It quietly adds protein, fiber, and omega-3 fats without changing the flavor much.

Bone Broth Grains

Cook rice, quinoa, or small pasta in bone broth instead of water. This adds protein and collagen to a familiar side dish with no extra steps once the broth is on hand.

The "No-Naked-Carb" Rule

Instead of serving carbs alone (crackers, pretzels, plain fruit), "dress" them with protein or fat:

- Apple slices with nut butter
- Crackers with cheese or hummus
- Banana with peanut butter
- Tortilla chips with guacamole or bean dip

This helps keep blood sugar steady, which prevents the immune system from being weakened by sudden sugar spikes.

Real-Life Plates: From Breakfast to Dinner

Families often ask me for simple, real-world examples. I am a pediatrician, not a chef, but there are a few patterns I come back to again and again.

Breakfast: "Power the Morning"

For kids, I am not a fan of the adult trend of skipping breakfast. Their brains and bodies need fuel early. A strong breakfast might look like a hard-boiled egg, a small bowl of plain yogurt, and a handful of blueberries for antioxidants. Oats can be helpful, especially for kids or parents needing help with cholesterol, but I use them sparingly and focus more on protein plus fruit to start the day.

Lunch: The Bento Box Approach

For school lunches, I like bento-style boxes with several small portions instead of one big item. A simple rule of thumb is to use your child's fist—not yours—as a serving guide: two "fists" of carbohydrates, one fist of protein, and one fist of healthy fat across the meal. In practice, that might be sliced cucumbers and carrots with hummus for dipping, a small portion of turkey or chicken, some peanut or nut butter (if allowed at school), and a section filled with berries or other fruit. Kids love to dip; if you give them something colorful to dip into, they are often more adventurous than you think.

Snacks and Dinner

After school, many kids come home starving. Rather than cookies or chips, I like to "reuse" the bento idea: more cut-up vegetables, fruit, hummus or nut butter, maybe some leftover chicken. Dinner can then focus on a good portion of protein, such as fish or chicken, plus vegetables like broccoli or broccolini and a smaller serving of rice or other grains. Even though kids need more carbohydrates than adults, I often suggest saving the bigger protein for dinner, when the family is together and more likely to sit down to a cooked meal.

Foods look different around the world. Where I live, strawberries and blueberries are common, but in other places, mango, papaya, watermelon, pineapple, or coconuts are everyday fruits. The main idea is to use local, affordable, and familiar foods to add color and variety to your child's plate. Lime can replace lemon, and local greens can replace spinach. You don't need to buy imported "superfoods" to give your child a healthy meal.

5. The "Sugar Swap": Strengthening Defenses Without Banning Treats

Sugar in large amounts can temporarily impair white blood cell function. You don't need to ban treats, but upgrading them can protect immunity while still letting kids enjoy something sweet.

The goal is to keep treats fun while quietly raising their nutritional value.

Instead of...	**Try...**
Fruit snacks (gummies)	Freeze-dried fruit (crunchy, naturally sweet)
Sweetened yogurt	Plain Greek yogurt with a drizzle of honey or fruit
Soda or full-strength juice	Sparkling water with a splash of 100% juice
Milk chocolate bar	Dark chocolate chips (around 70% cocoa) with almonds
Sugary granola bar	Homemade "energy balls" (dates, nuts, seeds, cocoa)

6. Supplement Dosage Guide: Ages & Stages

This is a general reference; always confirm doses with your child's provider.

Vitamin D3 (Typical Maintenance)

- Infants (0–12 months): 400 IU daily
- Toddlers (1–3 years): 600 IU daily
- School Age (4–8 years): 600–1,000 IU daily
- Older Children (9+ years): 1,000–2,000 IU daily

Children with known deficiencies may need different doses under medical supervision.

Zinc (Elemental)

For short-term "acute" support (up to about 5 days), unless your provider recommends otherwise:

- Toddlers (1–3 years): ~3 mg daily maintenance; 5–7 mg short-term
- School Age (4–8 years): ~5 mg daily maintenance; 10 mg short-term
- Older Children (9+ years): ~10 mg daily maintenance; 15–20 mg short-term

Always give with food and avoid prolonged high-dose use without guidance.

Vitamin C (Short-Term Support)

- Toddlers (1–3 years): up to ~250 mg/day, divided
- School Age (4–8 years): up to ~500 mg/day, divided

- Older Children (9+ years): 500–1,000 mg/day, divided

If loose stools develop, lower the dose.

7. Picky Eaters: Progress Over Perfection

If your child only eats beige foods and resists anything new, you are not failing. Picky eating is common, especially in early childhood, and forcing often backfires.

Helpful approaches:

- Keep offering small tastes of colorful foods without pressure.
- Model eating a rainbow yourself.
- Use "quiet nutrition" like power sprinkles, blended veggies in sauces, and bone-broth cooking water.
- Ask your pediatrician if a basic children's multivitamin is appropriate as a safety net.

I also see kids at the other end of the spectrum: children whose growth charts are two or three standard deviations above the curve with very high triglycerides or cholesterol. In those cases, we start with the same foundation—education, adjusting portions, swapping processed foods for whole foods—and, in a small number of cases, we add targeted supports like red yeast rice or even statins in the teenage years when genetically necessary. It is almost always easier to help a child gain healthy weight than to help them lose it later, which is why I am so passionate about building good habits early.

The goal is to make steady progress, not to have a perfect plate every time.

Nutrition is a quiet but powerful way to support your child's immune system every day. You don't need perfect meals or complicated recipes. Just add more color to their plate, make a few smart swaps for sugary snacks, keep them hydrated, and use a few well-chosen supplements when needed. These small, consistent choices give your child's body what it needs to stay strong and recover when they get sick.

In my clinic, I see the benefits of these choices over years, not just days. Some kids miss fewer school days, some teens recover faster from the same virus that keeps their friends home, and some families stop needing urgent care every winter. Food won't make your child invincible, but it can make them more resilient.

In the next chapter, we'll go beyond food and talk about the other side of immune health: movement, sleep, and stress. How your child moves, rests, and recovers affects how well their body uses the food you give them. We'll cover topics like screen time, sleep, outdoor play, sports, and simple ways to help your child's nervous system relax so their immune system can work well.

If nutrition is the supply line for your child's defenses, Chapter five is about the daily habits that help them use that fuel.

REFERENCES

Autier, P., Mullie, P., Macacu, A., Dragomir, M., Boniol, M., Coppens, K., Pizot, C., & Boniol, M. (2021). Screening for vitamin D deficiency in adults: Updated evidence report and systematic review for the US Preventive Services Task Force. JAMA, 325(14), 1443–1463. *https://doi.org/10.1001/jama.2020.26498*

Belkaid, Y., & Hand, T. W. (2014). Role of the microbiota in immunity and inflammation. Cell, 157(1), 121–141. *https://doi.org/10.1016/j.cell.2014.03.011*

Hawkins, J., Baker, C., Cherry, L., & Dunne, E. (2019). Black elderberry (Sambucus nigra) supplementation effectively treats upper respiratory symptoms: A meta-analysis of randomized, controlled clinical trials. Complementary Therapies in Medicine, 42, 361–365. *https://doi.org/10.1016/j.ctim.2018.12.004*

Hao, Q., Dong, B. R., & Wu, T. (2015). Probiotics for preventing acute upper respiratory tract infections. Cochrane Database of Systematic Reviews, 2015(2), CD006895. *https://doi.org/10.1002/14651858.CD006895.pub3*

Hewison, M. (2011). Vitamin D and innate and adaptive immunity. Vitamins and Hormones, 86, 23–62. *https://doi.org/10.1016/B978-0-12-386960-9.00002-2*

Mayo-Wilson, E., Junior, J. A., Imdad, A., Dean, S., Chan, X. H., Chan, E. S., Jaswal, A., & Bhutta, Z. A. (2014). Zinc supplementation for preventing mortality, morbidity, and growth failure in children aged 6 months to 12 years of age. Cochrane Database of Systematic Reviews, 2014(5), CD009384. *https://doi.org/10.1002/14651858.CD009384.pub2*

Pludowski, P., Takacs, I., Boyanov, M., Belaya, Z., Diaconu, C. C., Mokhort, T., Zherdova, N., Rasa, I., Payer, J., & Pilz, S. (2024). Vitamin D for the prevention of disease: An Endocrine Society clinical practice guideline. The Journal of Clinical Endocrinology and Metabolism, 109(8), 1823–1846. *https://doi.org/10.1210/clinem/dgae290*

Prasad, A. S. (2008). Zinc in human health: Effect of zinc on immune cells. Molecular Medicine, 14(5–6), 353–357. *https://doi.org/10.2119/2008-00033.Prasad*

Roschek, B., Jr., Fink, R. C., McMichael, M. D., Li, D., & Alberte, R. S. (2009). Elderberry flavonoids bind to and prevent H1N1 infection in vitro. Phytochemistry, 70(10), 1255–1261. *https://doi.org/10.1016/j.phytochem.2009.06.003*

Science, M., Johnstone, J., Roth, D. E., Guyatt, G., & Loeb, M. (2012). Zinc for the treatment of the common cold: A systematic review and meta-analysis of randomized controlled trials. CMAJ, 184(10), E551–E561. *https://doi.org/10.1503/cmaj.111990*

Szajewska, H., Hojsak, I., Kolacek, S., Orel, R., Shomarova, D., Tindberg, Y., Weizman, Z., & Vandenplas, Y. (2016). Probiotics for the prevention of antibiotic-associated diarrhea in children. Journal of Pediatric Gastroenterology and Nutrition, 62(3), 495–506. *https://doi.org/10.1097/MPG.0000000000001012*

Zakay-Rones, Z., Thom, E., Wollan, T., & Wadstein, J. (2004). Randomized study of the efficacy and safety of oral elderberry extract in the treatment of influenza A and B virus infections. Journal of International Medical Research, 32(2), 132–140. *https://doi.org/10.1177/147323000403200205*

CHAPTER 5

MOVEMENT, SLEEP & STRESS MANAGEMENT

The light flickered at 9:30 p.m., but ten-year-old Maya was still bouncing off the walls, picking fights with her little brother, and arguing about the math homework that wasn't even due until Friday. Her mom, Sarah, was exhausted.

"She used to be such a calm kid," Sarah told a friend. "Now, every day feels like a struggle. She's tired but won't settle down. She gets upset over little things and has had three colds in two months. I've tried cutting out sugar, adding a vitamin, and we even started reading at bedtime. Nothing helps. I feel like I'm missing the real problem."

Many parents today feel pressured to find complicated or expensive solutions for every problem, from a child's bad mood to a lingering cough. We often search online for the perfect supplement, the latest academic program, or a special after-school activity.

But what if the answer isn't to add something new, but to return to the basics that have always mattered most?

With busy family schedules, sleep, movement, and stress management often get pushed aside for homework, chores, and screen time. But these are actually the main things that keep a child's body healthy. Even the best nutrition can't do its job without them.

If you, like Sarah, have noticed that your child "just isn't themselves anymore," the answer may not be a complex diagnosis, but a quiet, powerful return to the basics. This chapter is about how to rebuild those foundations, transforming your child's health, mood, and resilience one good night's sleep and one burst of active play at a time.

Sleep and play are often treated as "extras" in a busy family schedule, squeezed in after homework, activities, and screens. Biologically, though, they are essential phases of immune maintenance. Active play boosts circulation and lymphatic flow, helping immune cells move throughout the body. Deep sleep triggers the release of cytokines, proteins that help fight infection and calm inflammation.

Nutrition, as c overed in Chapter four, gives your child fuel, but sleep, movement, and stress management are what keep things working. Without these, even a great diet can't fully protect your child. Like a car that needs regular use to stay in shape, the body needs movement, good sleep, and stress relief. The immune system's "training camp" from Chapter 1 also relies on these basics: sleep helps the immune system remember, movement keeps cells moving, and stress relief prevents the body from being overwhelmed.

Since COVID, I've seen how quickly these basics can fall apart. Many kids went from regular sports and school routines to long days indoors, late-night gaming, and little structure. Parents often say, "He just isn't himself anymore." We usually find poor sleep, little movement, and hidden stress. When we start to rebuild routines, even small changes can lead to big improvements in mood, health, and lab results.

A boy in my practice, about ten or twelve, came in for a checkup after missing visits during COVID. He used to be active, but now he had gained a lot of weight, had a big belly, and dark skin on his neck—signs of insulin resistance. His blood tests showed high cholesterol, high triglycerides, abnormal liver enzymes, and even prediabetes. He stayed up late gaming, slept in, skipped school, and barely moved from his bed to his screen. His parents were exhausted and felt stuck. In this chapter, I'll share the tools we used with him and other families to bring back movement, sleep, and a sense of control—without shame or needing to be perfect.

1. Sleep: The Recovery Engine

Sleep is not something we "fit in" if there's time. It is the body's built-in repair window and cannot be replaced by shortcuts. For kids, it supports growth, learning, mood regulation, and immune function.

During deep sleep, the immune system releases cytokines, specific proteins that help target infection and reduce inflammation. When children do not get enough sleep, their bodies make fewer of these protective proteins and have less reserve to fight off viruses.

The "Sleep Debt" Danger

Chronic sleep deprivation keeps the body in a low-grade inflammatory state. Over time, this makes children more vulnerable to frequent infections, especially in shared spaces like classrooms and daycare, where germs spread easily.

Target Sleep Totals (in 24 Hours)

These ranges include naps where appropriate:

- Toddlers (1–2 years): 11–14 hours
- Preschoolers (3–5 years): 10–13 hours
- School-age children (6–13 years): 9–11 hours
- Teens (14–17 years): 8–10 hours

Some kids land on the higher end of the range, others on the lower; the key is how they function during the day - energy, mood, and focus matter more than a perfect number.

The "Wind-Down" Protocol

When your child struggles to fall or stay asleep, it helps to think in terms of biology, not willpower. Three areas matter most: light, temperature, and routine.

Blue light restriction

Screens (phones, tablets, TVs, gaming systems) emit blue light, which signals to the brain that it is daytime and suppresses melatonin, the hormone that signals sleep. Aim to turn screens off at least one hour before bed and switch to calm, screen-free activities instead.

Cool, comfortable room

Most kids sleep best in a cool room, about 65-68°F. A small drop in body temperature tells the brain it's time to sleep. Lightweight pajamas and breathable bedding help, and a warm bath before bed followed by a cool room can make this drop more noticeable.

Predictable routine

A simple, repeatable routine, such as bath, pajamas, brush teeth, story, and song, helps the brain and body recognize, "Now we're going to sleep." Consistency is more important than complexity. Even on weekends, try to keep bedtime and wake time within about an hour of your weekday pattern.

How We Used Structure to Rescue Sleep

With the post-COVID gamer I mentioned earlier, we started by rebuilding sleep. Together with his family and school, we created a clear "contract": bedtime and wake time, no gaming after a set hour, and a requirement that he attend school (with a 504 plan providing some flexibility as he adjusted). We moved the gaming console out of his bedroom into a shared space so that playing became a visible, limited activity rather than an all-night habit. It was not quick or easy, and there were plenty of hard nights, but over time, his sleep normalized and his days stopped bleeding into his nights. That alone began to change his labs and his energy.

2. Movement: Keeping the Immune System in Motion

The heart circulates blood; the lymphatic system does not have its own pump. Instead, it relies on muscle movement and gravity to push lymph fluid through a network of vessels and nodes. That fluid carries immune cells, removes waste, and helps the body respond to infection. Long stretches of sitting can leave this system sluggish.

Regular movement in childhood is not just about "burning energy." It is a way to keep the immune system, brain, and mood in healthy motion.

"Play as Medicine"

Rebounding (jumping)

Jumping activities—on a mini-trampoline, a backyard trampoline with safety measures, or even repeated sets of jumping jacks—are especially effective for stimulating lymphatic flow. The gentle up-and-down shifts in gravity help open and close lymphatic valves, moving fluid along and giving immune cells a ride.

"Floor is Lava" games.

Homemade obstacle courses, crawling under tables, climbing over couch cushions, bear walks, crab walks, and rolling across the floor all engage large muscle groups. This full-body movement helps move lymph from the extremities back to the core and gives kids a fun way to be active indoors, especially in bad weather.

Aim for at least 60 minutes of active play a day, broken into smaller chunks (10–15 minutes at a time) if needed, rather than one long workout.

Green Exercise

Playing outside gives kids two big benefits: they move their bodies and spend time in nature. Being in green spaces like parks, backyards, or trails is linked to better mood, less stress, and a stronger immune system. Forest air has natural plant compounds (phytoncides) that may help immune cells fight viruses and even early cancer cells. Touching soil and being in nature also exposes kids to harmless microbes that help train their immune system. You don't need a wilderness trip—local parks, schoolyards, or backyards work too. The main thing is regular, unstructured time outside where kids can move, explore, and get fresh air.

What Changed for the "Gamer Kid"

For that ten-to-twelve-year-old boy, we did not start with a punishing workout plan. Once sleep and screen limits were in place, simply having less gaming time got him up and moving around the house more. Later, he picked up swimming at the local YMCA two or three times a week—nothing extreme. A year later, his weight had plateaued instead of climbing, his body shape had shifted away from visceral belly fat, his cholesterol and triglycerides had improved, and he was no longer prediabetic. The lab numbers mattered, but what I remember most is that he walked into the room more open, more willing to talk, and clearly more comfortable in his own skin. Movement and structure gave him that.

3. Stress Management: The Cortisol Connection

Children, like adults, feel stress, even if they don't have the words to describe it. Common stressors include loud or chaotic classrooms, a new sibling, academic pressure, friend conflicts, moves, illness in the family, or simply sensing parental worry.

The body's stress response releases cortisol and adrenaline. In short bursts, this can help us respond to challenges. But when cortisol stays high for long periods, it suppresses parts of the immune system and makes it harder to fight infections.

Signs of Stress in Kids

Kids rarely say, "I feel stressed." Instead, stress tends to show up in behavior and body symptoms, such as:

- Regression, such as bedwetting, clinginess, or tantrums over small things
- More frequent emotional outbursts or big reactions to minor frustrations
- Trouble falling asleep or staying asleep
- More headaches, stomachaches, nausea, or fatigue without a clear medical cause
- Changes in appetite or eating patterns
- Difficulty focusing, forgetfulness, or a drop in school performance
- Withdrawal from activities they usually enjoy, or more irritability and "attitude."

If these signs last more than a few weeks or start to affect daily life, it's a good idea to talk to your child's healthcare provider.

KID-FRIENDLY DE-STRESS TOOLS

"Blow Out the Candles" breathing. Have your child hold up one hand and imagine each finger is a candle. Inhale slowly through the nose, then blow out each "candle" with a long, gentle exhale through the mouth. Repeat until all the candles are "out." This type of slow breathing stimulates the vagus nerve and helps shift the body from "fight or flight" into "rest and digest."

Weighted blankets and deep pressure. Deep, even pressure on the body, like a firm hug, can increase calming neurotransmitters and lower cortisol. A child-appropriate weighted blanket, or simply snuggling under a stack of regular blankets, may help some kids feel more grounded and ready to sleep. Always choose a weight and size recommended for your child's age and body, and make sure they can move and breathe comfortably.

Aromatherapy: Scents for Calm and Comfort

Aromatherapy uses scent to influence the limbic system, the brain's emotional center. Smells travel directly from the nose to this part of the brain, which is why certain scents can quickly calm or uplift.

Used carefully, essential oils can be one tool among many to support your child's emotional regulation.

Lavender (the sedative)

Use: Diffuse in the bedroom for about 30 minutes before bedtime, or add a couple of drops to Epsom salts in a warm bath.

Effect: Lavender has been associated with lower heart rate and blood pressure and can promote deeper, more restful sleep.

Bergamot or sweet orange (the uplifters)

Use: On tough days, after school meltdowns, sibling conflicts, or emotional afternoons, diffuse in the kitchen or play area for a short period.

Effect: Citrus oils are known for their bright, mood-lifting properties and may help ease mild anxiety.

Roman chamomile (the soother)

Use: For general calming or to support teething comfort.

Application: Dilute one drop in about 1 tablespoon of carrier oil (such as coconut or jojoba) and gently massage it into the feet or along the spine.

Safety tips

- Always dilute essential oils for children; a common guideline is 0.5–1% dilution (about 1 drop of essential oil in 1–2 teaspoons of carrier oil), unless your provider advises otherwise.
- Do a small patch test on the skin to check for irritation.
- Avoid applying citrus oils on skin that will be in the sun, as they can increase sun sensitivity.
- Use age-appropriate oils; some oils are not recommended for babies or young children.
- Never let children ingest essential oils.

Parent Tip: The Oxygen Mask Rule

Children often act as emotional mirrors. They pick up on the tone of the home, the tension in our shoulders, and the speed of our voices. When caregivers are chronically stressed or anxious, kids can feel it, and their own stress response can stay activated.

The same rule you hear on airplanes applies here: put on your own oxygen mask before helping others. Taking care of your own stress isn't selfish—it's an important part of caring for your child, because your stress levels affect theirs.

MICRO-MOMENTS FOR PARENTS

You might not have time for long yoga classes or spa days, but small, regular moments of self-care can still make a real difference:

- Take 60 seconds of slow, deep breathing in the car before walking into the house after work.
- Do a brief stretch routine in the kitchen while something simmers on the stove.

- Step outside for a minute or two of fresh air and natural light between tasks.

- Keep a simple grounding habit, like feeling your feet on the floor and relaxing your shoulders, when you feel your own stress rising.

A calm parent sets the mood at home. When you feel steady, your child is more likely to feel steady too.

Key takeaway for parents: early recognition and support at home can make a big difference. A medical professional should evaluate ongoing or severe symptoms so your child can get the help they need.

Movement, sleep, and stress management aren't just extras—they're key to your child's immune health. Active play keeps immune cells moving. Deep, steady sleep lets the body repair and learn from each day. Simple ways to manage stress, for both you and your child, help keep cortisol in check so the immune system can work well. Along with good nutrition, these habits help your child handle the everyday germs they face.

The boy who walked into my office tired, heavy, and checked out after COVID did not become a different person overnight. But with clearer sleep boundaries, less screen time, a bit more movement, and adults who shared the load with him rather than fighting him, his body and confidence both began to heal. That is the kind of quiet, steady change these tools can offer your family, too.

Even with strong foundations in food, movement, sleep, and stress, the environment around your child still matters. The air they breathe, the way you clean, the bedding they sleep on, and even the fragrances in your home can either support or irritate their immune system.

In the next chapter, we will turn to the "home base" itself: air quality, strategic cleaning, decontamination routines, and safer choices for bedding and scents, so you can shape a home environment that quietly works with everything you are now doing for your child's health.

Chapter six will walk you through practical ways to tune that environment—managing pets and carpets, choosing gentler cleaners and soaps, and setting simple household routines—so the space your child lives in starts working with their immune system instead of against it.

Quick Guide: Parent Handout on Pediatric Stress

What is stress in children?

Stress is the body's response to changes or challenges. In children, it can come from school demands, family changes, peer issues, illness, sleep problems, or being overscheduled. Some stress is part of everyday life, but ongoing or intense stress can affect both physical and emotional health.

Common signs of stress

- Emotional: Irritability, frequent crying, worry, sadness, mood swings
- Behavioral: Withdrawal, aggression, regression (bedwetting, clinginess), changes in school performance
- Physical: Headaches, stomachaches, nausea, fatigue, changes in appetite
- Sleep: Trouble falling asleep, nightmares, frequent waking
- Attention: Difficulty focusing, forgetfulness

How parents can help at home

- Keep routines predictable (meals, bedtime, schoolwork).

- Encourage open conversations; listen and validate feelings.
- Model healthy coping (taking breaks, problem-solving calmly, asking for help).
- Support regular physical activity and adequate sleep.
- Protect downtime; avoid overscheduling.
- Monitor screen time and social media use.

When to call your child's healthcare provider

- Symptoms last more than 2–4 weeks or clearly worsen over time.
- Stress is interfering with school, sleep, or daily activities.
- Frequent physical complaints (stomachaches, headaches) without a clear cause.
- Noticeable changes in mood, behavior, or personality.
- Signs of anxiety or depression: persistent sadness, excessive worry, loss of interest in usual activities.
- Any talk of self-harm, feeling hopeless, or not wanting to be alive (seek urgent or emergency care immediately).

REFERENCES

Dempster, E. L., Pidsley, R., Schalkwyk, L. C., Owens, S., Georgiades, A., Kane, F., Kalidindi, S., Picchioni, M., Kravariti, E., Toulopoulou, T., Murray, R. M., & Mill, J. (2019). Intergenerational transmission of depression: Clinical observations and molecular mechanisms. Molecular Psychiatry, 24(9), 1240–1253. *https://doi.org/10.1038/s41380-018-0265-z*

Jaffee, S. R., & Arseneault, L. (2021). Editorial: The value of genetically informative designs to understand pathways of intergenerational transmission and direction of causality. Journal of the American Academy of Child and Adolescent Psychiatry, 60(4), 454–456. *https://doi.org/10.1016/j.jaac.2020.07.906*

Levy, O. (2015). Development of immunity in early life. The Journal of Infection, 71(Suppl. 1), S112–S115. *https://doi.org/10.1016/j.jinf.2015.04.027*

Principi, N., & Esposito, S. (2012). Principles of inflammation for the pediatrician. Pediatric Clinics of North America, 59(6), 1161–1171. *https://doi.org/10.1016/j.pcl.2012.08.001*

Shonkoff, J. P., Garner, A. S., & The Committee on Psychosocial Aspects of Child and Family Health, Committee on Early Childhood, Adoption, and Dependent Care, and Section on Developmental and Behavioral Pediatrics. (2021). Leveraging the biology of adversity and resilience to transform pediatric practice. Pediatrics, 147(2), e2020049437. *https://doi.org/10.1542/peds.2020-049437*

Viner, R., Russell, S., Saulle, R., Croker, H., Stansfield, C., Packer, J., Nicholls, D., Goddings, A.-L., Bonell, C., Hudson, L., Hope, S., Ward, J., Schwalbe, N., Morgan, A., & Minozzi, S. (2021). Immunity in the very young: Challenges and opportunities. Immunity, 49(4), 604–618. *https://doi.org/10.1016/j.immuni.2018.08.009*

Chapter 6

HOME ENVIRONMENT FOR HEALTH

Your child's body is their first defense against getting sick, and your home is the second. Earlier, we talked about what happens inside your child—how their immune system works, how fever and cough help them heal, and how things like food, movement, sleep, and stress play a role. Now, let's look at how these same ideas apply to the spaces, routines, and products your child uses every day.

In this chapter, we're focusing on your child's surroundings. The air they breathe, the things they touch, and even what's in their bedding all quietly affect how much work their immune system has to do.

This chapter isn't about making your home spotless or trying to get rid of every germ. A perfectly clean home isn't realistic or even good for your child's immune system. Instead, the goal is to lower the overall "toxic load"—the everyday irritants, chemicals, and germs your child's body deals with—using simple steps. That way, their immune system can focus on the germs that really matter.

Early in my career, I learned how much a child's home environment can matter. I once cared for a six- to seven-month-old baby with ongoing diarrhea—not just loose stools, but watery with mucus and sometimes blood. We tried the usual things: changing the breastfeeding parent's diet, adding probiotics, and using foods like bananas and yogurt. Each time, the problem got better for a bit, then came back. The baby never seemed very sick and didn't have fevers, but the pattern kept repeating. Eventually, we tested the stool and found unusual bacteria, which made me wonder, "What's happening at home?" When standard treatments only helped for a short time, it was a sign that something in the environment was causing the problem. That question is what this chapter is all about.

1. Air Quality: The Invisible Immune Suppressor

The Environmental Protection Agency says indoor air can be two to five times more polluted than outdoor air. Modern, tightly sealed homes save energy, but they can also trap germs, carbon dioxide, and allergens inside.

"Dilution is the Solution"

Fresh air is one of the simplest tools you have.

- Open windows for about 10–15 minutes each morning, when the weather allows, even in winter.
- This quick air exchange helps flush out stale, virus-laden air and brings in fresh, oxygen-rich air.

You don't have to keep the house chilly; even a brief daily "airing out" makes a difference. If you live near heavy traffic, industrial sites, or wildfire smoke, check local air quality first and skip window time on poor-air days.

The "Goldilocks" Humidity Zone

Viruses and our airways behave differently depending on how dry or damp the air is.

- Dry air (below about 30% humidity): Viruses like influenza and COVID-19 can linger longer and spread more easily in very dry air. Dry air also dries out the lining of your child's nose, making it harder for them to trap germs.

- Damp air (above about 60% humidity): Too much moisture encourages mold and dust mites, which are common triggers for allergies and asthma.

Aim for a "just right" humidity between about 40% and 60%. As a quick thumb-rule, if the windows fog up frequently, it's likely too damp. On the other hand, if your skin or lips feel excessively dry, the air might be too dry. These sensory cues can guide you even if you don't have a hygrometer handy.

- Use a small hygrometer (humidity meter) to check levels.
- In winter, a cool-mist humidifier can raise humidity.
- In damp seasons or basements, a dehumidifier can bring it down.

Whichever device you use, clean it regularly according to the instructions; dirty humidifiers or filters can themselves become sources of mold or bacteria.

Bedroom Air: Where They Spend Half Their Life

Your child spends a huge portion of their life in their bedroom, especially when they are sick.

- Consider using a standalone HEPA air purifier in their room.
- HEPA filters can remove very small particles, including dust, pet dander, and some airborne germs, reducing the burden on your child's lungs while they sleep.

You don't need to buy an expensive whole-house system. Having one air purifier that fits the bedroom is a good start. If that's not possible, regular dusting, vacuuming with a HEPA bag if you can, and opening windows when the air is good are still helpful.

2. Kid-Proofing Against Germs: Strategic Cleaning

You don't need to clean your whole house every day. The important thing is to focus on the places where germs are most likely to spread between people.

High-Touch Surfaces: The Real "Super-Spreaders"

Floors are often cleaned regularly, even though kids rarely get sick from walking across them. Meanwhile, the true "super-spreader" spots are easy to miss:

- Light switches
- Doorknobs
- Remote controls and gaming controllers
- Refrigerator and microwave handles
- Faucet handles and toilet flush levers

During cold and flu season:

- Wipe these high-touch surfaces once a day (or as often as you reasonably can) with a safe cleaner or disinfectant. Many respiratory viruses can survive on hard plastic surfaces for up to 24–48 hours, which makes regular cleaning an important layer of protection.
- This targeted approach takes just a few minutes and reduces the number of germs that move from hands to faces. Day to day, a simple soap-based cleaner is often enough; save stronger disinfectants for when someone at home is actively sick.

The Toothbrush Trap

Bathrooms are humid, and toothbrushes often end up stored together in a cup with their heads touching.

- Keep toothbrushes standing up and make sure the bristles don't touch each other.

- After strep throat, a stomach bug, or other significant infection, replace your child's toothbrush to reduce the chance of re-exposure. If replacing isn't possible right away, rinsing well and letting the brush dry completely between uses is still helpful.

3. Family Routines: A Simple "Decontamination" Protocol

Schools, daycares, and playgrounds are full of germs. You can't (and shouldn't) avoid them completely. What you *can* do is set up a simple routine that stops as many germs as possible at the door.

The "Shoes Off" Rule

Shoes bring in more than just dirt. They can carry lawn chemicals, road dust, and bacteria from public restrooms and sidewalks into your home.

- Get everyone, including adults, in the habit of taking off their shoes at the door.

- Put a bin or shoe rack by the door to make it easy for everyone.

Clothes Change and Handwashing

Clothes worn in classrooms and daycares pick up germs all day.

A simple after-school routine:

- Come in the door.

- Shoes off.

- Wash hands with soap and water for about 20 seconds, which is about as long as it takes to sing "Happy Birthday."
- Change out of school clothes and put on clean clothes for home.

Help kids stick to the routine by making it easy:

- Use a sturdy step stool so they can reach the sink.
- Choose a fun, foaming soap or one with a scent they like.
- Hang a small hook or basket for "school clothes," so they don't end up on the couch or bed.

This isn't about being perfect. Even doing these steps most days makes a big difference in what comes into your home. On tough nights, just getting the handwashing done still helps.

I remember one night when everyone was running late, dinner was a mismatch of leftovers, and bedtime was looming. Chaos reigned, but we made sure hands were washed. That's the reality of parenting—embracing the imperfect moments while still taking small steps for health.

What We Found in the Baby's Home

When I went back to that six-month-old with chronic diarrhea and the strange bacteria on the stool test, I asked the parents more about their home. That is when they mentioned their pet iguanas. Iguanas, like many reptiles, can carry bacteria such as E. coli and Pseudomonas. These pets were allowed to roam and occasionally urinate or defecate on the carpet without anyone noticing. Once the baby started crawling, he was right down on that same carpet, putting his hands and toys into his mouth. That was the missing piece. We worked with the family to confine the iguanas to specific, easy-to-clean areas and to keep the baby off those floors. Once we separated the baby from the invisible "pet zones" and tightened up cleaning in those areas, his diarrhea resolved. The lesson was not "never have pets," but "know where they go" and keep babies' play spaces clean and separate whenever possible. The same principle applies to cat litter boxes, dog accidents, and any area where animals eat or eliminate. Sometimes the most powerful "treatment" isn't a new medicine at all—it's moving the source.

4. Cleaning Products and Fragrance: Reducing Irritants

Many conventional cleaning products and air fresheners contain strong chemicals that can irritate the airways, especially in children with asthma or allergies. When the respiratory system is constantly irritated, the immune system may be more easily triggered by otherwise minor exposures.

"Fragrance" on the Label

When you see "fragrance" or "parfum" on an ingredient list, it usually means a mix of many chemicals. Some of these can irritate or disrupt hormones.

Simple swaps:

- Choose unscented versions of laundry detergents, cleaners, and fabric softeners when possible.
- If you like scents, look for products scented with clearly listed essential oils, not "fragrance blends."
- Avoid plug-in air fresheners and heavy room sprays; try opening windows, using an air purifier, or simmering spices (like cinnamon sticks) on the stove for scent instead. Even natural scents can bother some kids, so start small and watch how your child does.

Safer Cleaning Basics

You don't need a separate product for every surface.

- Glass/surface cleaner: A 50/50 mix of water and white vinegar works for many surfaces (avoid on natural stone like marble).
- Disinfectant: Hydrogen peroxide (the standard 3% solution sold in brown bottles) can be a gentler alternative to bleach for many household disinfection needs; it breaks down into water and oxygen after use.

Always keep cleaning products where children can't reach them.

How I Think About Cleaners at Home

Personally, I grew up loving the smell of bleach because it reminded me of hospitals, and made me feel "clean." Over time, though, I have learned that we can get a lot of the cleaning benefit without so many harsh fumes. At home, I still use stronger disinfectants when needed, but for everyday wiping and mopping, I lean on basics like diluted vinegar, hydrogen peroxide, and simple soaps. They reduce the chemical load in the house while still getting the job done. It's another place where progress, not perfection, makes a real difference.

5. Soap, Skin, and Everyday Products

It is not just what you clean the house with; it is also what you clean your child with. In my own family, when I worked in the emergency department, we had a simple routine: when we came home, our outer clothes went straight into a laundry basket by the door, and we headed to the bathroom to shower. Our go-to was plain Castile soap, a basic soap made from oils that cleans well without a long list of additives. We often added a few drops of essential oils like lemon, lavender, or peppermint (always well diluted) for scent and the mild antimicrobial properties they provide.

Handwashing still matters more than any fancy product. COVID-19 taught us again that washing with plain soap and water and using friction dramatically lowers viral load on the hands. You do not need antibacterial soap. In fact, the old antibacterial additives in many soaps killed helpful bacteria on the skin and have largely fallen out of favor. Plain soap and water, and 20 seconds of rubbing, are enough. If "Happy Birthday" has worn out its welcome, choose any short song or chorus your child enjoys and use that instead.

How often you bathe your child and what moisturizers you use are also part of the home environment. Different cultures have different bathing habits. As long as your child's skin isn't breaking down, infected, or very itchy, you're probably doing fine. Bathing too often, especially with harsh soaps, can remove natural oils and make skin dry and more likely to get irritated. For moisturizing, simple oils like coconut, avocado, or olive oil, or products rich in oleic acid, can work just as well—and are often safer and cheaper—than many baby creams. I'm more careful with trendy products like beef-tallow balms because they're animal-based and not as well studied in kids, especially those with allergies. In most cases, good-quality plant oils give you similar benefits with fewer unknowns.

6. Bedding: The Dust Mite Defense

If your child wakes up with a stuffy nose or itchy eyes that get better later in the day, dust mites in their bedding might be the cause. Dust mites love pillows and mattresses, and their waste can trigger allergies.

Simple bedding routine:

- Wash sheets and pillowcases in hot water (at least 130°F) about once a week. Hot water kills dust mites, while cold water mostly just removes dirt.

- Consider allergen-proof covers for pillows and mattresses, especially if your child has allergies or asthma.

- Wash the pillows themselves (not just the cases) every 3-6 months, following the label instructions. If you can't wash them, replace them from time to time.

You don't have to overhaul everything at once. Even one change, like adding an allergen-proof pillow cover, can make mornings more comfortable. If covers aren't accessible right now, even washing bedding more often can still help.

Movement, sleep, and stress (from Chapter five) are the "software" your child's immune system runs on day to day. Your home environment is the "hardware" it runs in. Small changes to air quality, cleaning routines, handwashing, and bedding can quietly lower the background strain on your child's body, so their immune system is freer to do what it does best: respond to real infections and then stand down. You do not need to change everything at once; even one small tweak in either the "hardware" or the "software" still counts.

The baby with chronic diarrhea did not need a rare medication; he needed us to see what was happening on his living room floor. Once we changed the environment under his hands and knees, his gut settled down. That is the power of looking beyond the body to the space it lives in.

In the next chapter, we'll take these ideas beyond your front door—to schools, sports, and the wider community settings where your child spends so much of their time. With the tools you have collected so far, you are building not just a healthier child, but a calmer, more confident home base for your whole family.

REFERENCES

Bocchini, J. A., Jr., & Garfunkel, L. C. (2020). Pediatric prevention: General prevention. Pediatric Clinics of North America, 67(2), 267–280. *https://doi.org/10.1016/j.pcl.2019.12.001*

Brady, M. T., Byington, C. L., Davies, H. D., Edwards, K. M., Frenck, R. W., Jr., Gerber, M. A., Jackson, M. A., Kehl, S. C., Murray, D. L., Lynfield, R., Nigrovic, L. E., Nyquist, A.-C., Rathore, M. H., Saez-Llorens, X., Schwartz, B., Tanus, T., & Zaoutis, T. E. (2017). Infection prevention and control in pediatric ambulatory settings. Pediatrics, 140(5), e20172857. *https://doi.org/10.1542/peds.2017-2857*

Conly, J., & Johnston, B. (2011). Hygiene: New hopes, new horizons. The Lancet Infectious Diseases, 11(1), 2–3. *https://doi.org/10.1016/S1473-3099(10)70261-6*

Cumming, O., Arnold, B. F., Ban, R., Clasen, T., Esteves Mills, J., Freeman, M. C., Gordon, B., Guiteras, R., Howard, G., Hunter, P. R., Johnston, R. B., Pickering, A. J., Prakash, M., Prüss-Ustün, A., Schmidt, W.-P., Shin, G. A., Trinies, V., & Wolf, J. (2019). The implications of three major new trials for the effect of water, sanitation and hygiene on childhood diarrhea and stunting: A consensus statement. BMC Medicine, 17(1), 173. *https://doi.org/10.1186/s12916-019-1381-x*

Ejemot-Nwadiaro, R. I., Ehiri, J. E., Meremikwu, M. M., & Critchley, J. A. (2020). Hand cleaning with ash for reducing the spread of viral and bacterial infections: A rapid review. Cochrane Database of Systematic Reviews, 2020(4), CD013597. *https://doi.org/10.1002/14651858.CD013597*

McDonald, L. C., Gerding, D. N., Johnson, S., Bakken, J. S., Carroll, K. C., Coffin, S. E., Dubberke, E. R., Garey, K. W., Gould, C. V., Kelly, C., Loo, V., Sammons, J. S., Sandora, T. J., & Wilcox, M. H. (2018). Clinical practice guidelines for Clostridium difficile infection in adults and children: 2017 update by the Infectious Diseases Society of America (IDSA) and Society for Healthcare Epidemiology of America (SHEA). Clinical Infectious Diseases, 66(7), e1–e48. *https://doi.org/10.1093/cid/cix1085*

Milstone, A. M., Maragakis, L. L., & Perl, T. M. (2024). SHEA practice update: Infection prevention and control (IPC) in residential facilities for pediatric patients and their families.

Infection Control and Hospital Epidemiology, 45(1), 1–14. *https://doi.org/10.1017/ice.2023.231*

Yokoe, D. S., Anderson, D. J., Berenholtz, S. M., Calfee, D. P., Dubberke, E. R., Ellingson, K. D., Gerding, D. N., Haas, J. P., Kaye, K. S., Klompas, M., Lo, E., Marschall, J., Mermel, L. A., Nicolle, L. E., Salgado, C. D., Bryant, K., Classen, D., Crist, K., Deloney, V. M., … Calfee, D. P. (2010). Prevention of healthcare-associated infections in children: New strategies and success stories. Current Opinion in Infectious Diseases, 23(4), 372–379. *https://doi.org/10.1097/QCO.0b013e32833b7b46*

CHAPTER 7

SEASONAL FLU & BACK-TO-SCHOOL TIPS

Every parent knows that late-August feeling. Just as your family settles into the healthier rhythm of summer, more sun, more sleep, more outside time, the "Back-to-School" signs appear, and you can almost *feel* the germs lining up at the classroom door.

School brings structure and friends, but it also means long days indoors with many other children, shared supplies, and a steady stream of viruses. You can't protect your child from every germ, and you don't need to. What you *can* do is stack the odds in their favor. This chapter gives you practical, realistic routines to get through back-to-school and flu season with more confidence and fewer crises.

Every fall in my practice, I notice a pattern: families with kids in different schools suddenly dealing with lots of new germs. Surprisingly, it's often the teenager—who we think is the toughest—who gets the sickest. I once cared for a high schooler who ignored early flu symptoms, kept going to school while eating mostly chips and soda, and skipped the flu shot. When he finally came in, he had trouble breathing, a high fever, and blood tests showed anemia and low platelets. He needed hospital care for something that could have been much milder if we had supported his health and paid attention to his early symptoms. That's why I care so much about simple, layered protections before and during flu season.

1. THE "2-WEEK COUNTDOWN": RESETTING THE RHYTHM

The immune system works best with consistency. In Chapter five , we talked about how sleep and stress affect your child's resilience, and in Chapter four , we covered how nutrition supports their immune system. Switching from "summer mode" with late nights and random meals to "school mode" with early alarms and homework can be a real shock to their system.

That shock raises cortisol, the body's main stress hormone, and can temporarily weaken immune defenses, right when your child is suddenly sharing air and crayons with twenty other kids. Remember the kindergartner from Chapter one who had 17 viral illnesses in his first school year? A smoother transition into that new environment could not have prevented every illness, but it could have made some of those rounds easier on his body and his family.

The Sleep Shift

Instead of trying to fix bedtime the night before school starts, give everyone a gentle on-ramp.

- Two weeks before the first day, move bedtime earlier by about 15 minutes each night.
- At the same time, wake your child 15 minutes earlier each morning.

By the first day of school, your child should be able to wake up around their school start time without feeling like a zombie. A well-rested child handles both germs and emotions better; a sleep-deprived child is more likely to get sick and melt down.

Breakfast Training

Summer breakfasts often drift later and can be more "grab-what's-around."

- As you shift sleep, also shift breakfast back to the school-day hour.

- Aim for a breakfast with protein and healthy fat (eggs, yogurt, nut butter toast, leftovers) rather than just sugary cereal or pastries.

Sending your child to school on an empty stomach or only on sugar sets them up for a blood sugar crash mid-morning. That "crash" leaves them tired, cranky, and less able to maintain strong immune defenses.

2. The Classroom Survival Guide

Teachers work hard to keep classrooms clean and organized, but they are outnumbered. One of the best gifts you can give your child is a few simple, clear rules for protecting their own space and supplies.

Provide them with easy, polite scripts like, "No thank you, that's my bottle," or "I use my own things," which can empower them to manage their personal items and reduce how much you have to coach from the sidelines. These scripts help build consistency and self-advocacy.

The "No-Share" Rule (With an Asterisk)

We teach kids that sharing is kind, and that's still true. We just need to add an exception.

- Script it this way: "We share toys and ideas, but we **never** share food, drinks, or lip balm. That is how germs travel."

This keeps the spirit of generosity while quietly blocking some of the easiest paths for viruses and stomach bugs.

The Water Fountain Bypass

School water fountains are classic germ hubs.

- Send a sturdy, easy-to-open, clearly labeled water bottle every day.
- Teach your child that their bottle is their "personal fountain," and they don't need to put their mouth near the school spout.

Hand Sanitizer Etiquette

Soap and water are best, but they're not always available.

- Clip a small hand sanitizer to your child's backpack or lunchbox.
- Teach the "Rub until Dry" rule: pump, rub over all surfaces of the hands, and keep rubbing until no moisture remains. If hands are still wet, the sanitizer hasn't done its full job, and kids are more likely to wipe the alcohol into their eyes.

3. Flu Season Prep (October–March)

As days get shorter and the heat comes on, more viruses start to circulate in the community. This is a good time to strengthen the habits you've built around sleep, nutrition, and your home environment. That way, your child enters the season with as much protection as possible.

The Vitamin D Bump

By October, in many places, the sun is no longer strong enough for kids to make much Vitamin D from skin exposure, especially if they are inside most of the day.

- This is a key time to start or adjust Vitamin D supplementation, as discussed in Chapter four , under your child's provider's guidance.

- Steady Vitamin D support through fall and winter can help keep immune defenses ready.

The Humidifier Routine

Heated indoor air is often very dry, which dries out the nose and throat and makes it easier for viruses to take hold.

- Run a cool-mist humidifier in your child's bedroom at night during heating season, aiming for that 40–60% humidity "Goldilocks zone" you learned about in Chapter six.

- Clean the humidifier regularly according to the manufacturer's instructions so you're not blowing mold into the air.

Support the Teacher (and Your Child)

The cleaner the classroom, the healthier the kids.

- When you're able, donate tissues, wipes, and hand sanitizer to your child's classroom.

- A small contribution from many families can make a real difference in how often surfaces get wiped and noses get covered.

Layering Everyday Habits

In families like the one with my very sick teenager, I emphasize basics before school starts: real food instead of chips and soda, a regular bedtime, and enough water to support the body if a fever hits. I also encourage handwashing "bookends" before leaving for school, before and after lunch, after using the bathroom, and as soon as they get home. If someone in their class is clearly coughing and sick, I let my patients know it is okay to wear a mask. That is now a socially accepted layer of protection many teens and kids are comfortable with, especially in peak flu weeks.

4. Navigating the Flu Shot

The decision to vaccinate should always be made with your child's healthcare provider, taking your family's needs and values into account. If you choose the flu shot, a little planning can help your child's body respond well.

One helpful question is, "Will this protection still cover spring break travel?" Working backward from key dates can guide timing and make the decision feel more concrete.

- **Timing:** It typically takes about two weeks after the shot for antibodies to develop. For many families, mid-October is a "sweet spot" so protection lasts through the peak months (often January–February).

- **Don't stack stressors**: Whenever possible, avoid scheduling vaccines on days when your child is already ill, very overtired, or under a lot of stress. You want their immune system calm and ready to respond.

Day-of and after-care tips:

- Make sure they are well-hydrated and slept reasonably well the night before.

- Gentle arm movements or play that uses the vaccinated arm can reduce soreness.

- A warm bath with Epsom salts in the evening (if approved by your provider) can help with general post-shot achiness.

Why I Rarely Skip My Flu Shot

Personally, I cannot emphasize enough how important the flu shot has been for me. I have been getting a flu shot for decades. The one year I forgot, back in 2016, I became so ill that I was out of the clinic and flat on my back, thinking, "Never again." Since then, I have not missed it. For kids who are immunocompromised or have conditions like heart disease or diabetes, I strongly recommend the flu shot because the flu can be especially dangerous for them. For otherwise healthy kids, it is still a powerful layer of protection that can turn a potentially severe illness into a much milder one.

5. Supplements, Food, and Flu-Season Helpers

Parents are often overwhelmed by long lists of supplements. In my practice, I keep it simple: a high-quality multivitamin (or a whole-food concentrate like Juice Plus, if it fits your budget and preferences), plus a few targeted supports. Nutrient-dense foods rich in zinc (seeds, beans, lentils), vitamin C (citrus, mango, papaya, pineapple, berries), and anti-inflammatory spices like garlic and turmeric pull a lot of weight. I encourage families to build those into everyday meals, such as marinating chicken with turmeric, garlic, and onion, or simmering a simple chai-style tea with ginger, turmeric, cinnamon, and other spices. That way, immune support is baked into what you are already cooking, not one more "thing" to remember.

Garlic and turmeric provide antioxidant and antimicrobial support and can be easily added to soups, stews, roasted vegetables, and marinades.

Elderberry and Chamomile

Elderberry syrup is another tool I like for families. Research suggests elderberry may support a healthy immune response. Chamomile is often used to promote relaxation and may support sleep, which is central to immune defense. Elderberry, especially when combined with honey for kids over one year old, also acts as a mucolytic, which helps thin mucus so it is easier to clear.

I usually suggest using elderberry in short bursts: at the very start of cold and flu season, before a big exposure like the first week of school, or at the first hint of symptoms. Using it all year long can turn it into background noise instead of a true "boost."

Nasal and Throat Hygiene

Saline or xylitol nasal sprays and salt-water gargles are simple, low-cost tools that help rinse viruses and bacteria off the nasal and throat lining, especially after high-exposure days.

Vitamin D, Vitamin C, and Zinc

Vitamin D, covered in earlier chapters, is still essential for bone and immune health in fall and winter. Foods rich in vitamin C and, when needed, supplements can help the immune system, and zinc (from foods or short-term supplements) is important for fighting viruses. Always check the right dose with your child's provider.

Water: How Much and What Kind?

Staying hydrated is one of the most important but often overlooked tools during flu season. The main complication I worry about with the flu is dehydration, since high fevers make kids lose fluids quickly and they may not want to drink. As a general rule, I suggest about 2-3 ounces of fluid per pound of body weight per day for kids up to age two, and about 1-1.5 ounces per pound for older kids, adjusting for activity, climate, and medical advice. Your child's clinician can help you find the right amount for your child.

Quality matters too, but it does not have to be complicated or expensive. At my home in Long Beach, we are fortunate to have decent city water, and I use a three-stage under-sink filter (sediment, UV, then carbon) to remove particles, kill microbes, and improve taste. In areas with wells, septic systems, or questionable municipal water supply, families may need more robust filtration or storage systems, often with built-in settling tanks and disinfection. Local water reports are a helpful starting point. I am cautious about high-pH "alkaline" waters for kids; their kidneys are not as equipped as adults' to handle big pH swings, and they do not need softened or heavily buffered water with extra salts. Simple, well-filtered water in adequate amounts is the goal.

I am also not a big fan of reverse osmosis systems for most families because they waste a lot of water; only a small fraction of what goes in becomes drinking water, and the rest is discarded. If a family chooses reverse osmosis for specific reasons, I encourage them to find ways to reuse the wastewater, such as irrigation, when it is safe and allowed.

6. The "24-Hour Rule": When to Return to School

One of the biggest drivers of school outbreaks is kids going back too soon. As a parent, you juggle work, siblings, and logistics, and it can be tempting to send a "mostly better" child back as soon as a fever drops. But returning too early often backfires.

The Golden Fever Rule

- Your child should be fever-free for at least **24 hours without** fever-reducing medicine (like Acetaminophen or Ibuprofen) before going back.
- If the only thing holding the fever down is medication, the infection is still active, and they are still contagious.

Always check your school's specific policies, but this 24-hour guideline is a good baseline.

The Vomit/Diarrhea Rule

The same 24-hour principle applies to stomach bugs.

- Wait at least 24 hours after the last episode of vomiting or diarrhea before returning to school or daycare.
- Stomach viruses like norovirus are highly contagious, and sending a child back too soon can lead to rapid spread.

The Energy Check

Even if the fever is gone, ask yourself:

- Are they acting like themselves?
- Do they have the energy to get through a school day without crashing?

If your child is pale, very quiet, unusually clingy, or clearly wiped out, an extra "boring day" at home can prevent complications and relapse. That extra day lets their immune system finish what it started instead of being pushed back into the fray too soon.

7. Quick Year-Round Routines

A few small weekly habits can quietly break many germ chains.

- **The "high-five" reminder**: At drop-off, use a quick cue like, "High-five for washing hands before snack!" Kids often respond well to simple, positive prompts.
- **The Friday reset**: Once a week, Friday after school works well, do a mini clean of your child's "school gear":
- Wipe down backpack handles and zippers.
- Put the water bottle in the dishwasher (use the sanitize cycle if your dishwasher has one).
- Wipe or wash the lunchbox inside and out.
- Toss frequently used hats, gloves, or light jackets into the wash, especially in peak cold/flu season.

Parent Handout: Vitamin D Basics for Kids

You can adapt this as a one-page handout for families in your practice or community.

Why Vitamin D Matters

Vitamin D supports healthy bones, teeth, muscles, and immune function. Many children do not get enough from food and sunlight alone, so daily supplementation is often recommended.

Typical Daily Vitamin D Doses by Age (Always confirm with your child's clinician.)

- Birth–12 months: 400 IU (10 mcg) daily
- 1–12 years: 600 IU (15 mcg) daily
- 13–18 years: 600 IU (15 mcg) daily

Children with certain medical conditions, limited sun exposure, or higher body weight may need different dosing under medical supervision.

How to Give Vitamin D

- Infants: liquid vitamin D drops
- Children and teens: chewables, gummies, tablets, or liquid
- Can usually be taken with or without food, once per day

Safety Notes

- Do not exceed recommended doses unless your child's clinician specifically advises it.
- Store supplements out of reach; they are potent, not candies.
- Ask your provider which product and dose are best if your child has chronic conditions or takes daily medications.

Key Takeaway: Daily Vitamin D from infancy through adolescence is a simple, low-effort way to support long-term bone and immune health.

Back-to-school and flu season will never be completely germ-free, and that's okay. Your child's immune "library" grows every time they face and recover from an infection, just like the boy in Chapter one , whose 17 illnesses slowly turned into fewer, milder colds as his system learned. What you've done in the earlier chapters—supporting sleep, nutrition, stress, your home environment, and now school routines—gives their body a strong foundation.

Layering these logistical habits on top—smoother schedule transitions, classroom rules that protect without creating fear, smart flu-season routines, and thoughtful decisions about when to stay home—helps you move through the highest-risk months with more calm and fewer surprises. You can't control every virus in the classroom, but you *can* control the rhythms and routines that make your child more ready to face them.

In the final chapter, we will pull all of these pieces together—immune "training camp," fevers and coughs, food and supplements, sleep and stress, home environment, and school strategies—into a simple, realistic roadmap. The goal is not a perfect, germ-free childhood, but a resilient child and a calmer parent who both know what to do next time the sniffles, fevers, or school emails start rolling in.

REFERENCES

American Academy of Pediatrics Committee on Infectious Diseases. (2023). Recommendations for prevention and control of influenza in children, 2023–2024. Pediatrics, 152(4), e2023063737. *https://doi.org/10.1542/peds.2023-063737*

American Academy of Pediatrics Committee on Infectious Diseases. (2024). Recommendations for prevention and control of influenza in children, 2024–2025: Policy statement. Pediatrics, 154(4), e2024068508. *https://doi.org/10.1542/peds.2024-068508*

American Academy of Pediatrics Committee on Infectious Diseases. (2025). Recommendations for prevention and control of influenza in children, 2025–2026: Policy statement. Pediatrics, 155(4), e2025071049. *https://doi.org/10.1542/peds.2025-071049*

Cauchemez, S., Valleron, A.-J., Boelle, P.-Y., Flahault, A., & Ferguson, N. M. (2008). Estimating the impact of school closure on influenza transmission from sentinel data. Nature, 452(7188), 750–754. *https://doi.org/10.1038/nature06732*

Cowling, B. J., Lau, L. L. H., Wu, P., Wong, H. W. C., Fang, V. J., Riley, S., & Nishiura, H. (2013). Effect of winter school breaks on influenza-like illness, Argentina, 2005–2008. Emerging Infectious Diseases, 19(6), 938–944. *https://doi.org/10.3201/eid1906.121377*

Jefferson, T., Dooley, L., Ferroni, E., Al-Ansary, L. A., van Driel, M. L., Bawazeer, G. A., Jones, M. A., Hoffmann, T. C., Clark, J., Beller, E. M., Glasziou, P. P., & Conly, J. M. (2023). Physical interventions to interrupt or reduce the spread of respiratory viruses. Cochrane Database of Systematic Reviews, 2023(1), CD006207. *https://doi.org/10.1002/14651858.CD006207.pub6*

Krishnaratne, S., Pfadenhauer, L. M., Bjørnholt, J. V., Burns, J., Charoenwong, B., Chilcott, H., … Lorenc, T. (2022). Measures implemented in the school setting to contain the COVID-19 pandemic: A rapid review. Cochrane Database of Systematic Reviews, 2022(8), CD015029. *https://doi.org/10.1002/14651858.CD015029*

Prather, A. A., Janicki-Deverts, D., Hall, M. H., & Cohen, S. (2015). Behaviorally assessed sleep and susceptibility to the common cold. Sleep, 38(9), 1353–1359. *https://doi.org/10.5665/sleep.4968*

Wagner, C. L., & Greer, F. R. (2008). Prevention of rickets and vitamin D deficiency in infants, children, and adolescents. Pediatrics, 122(5), 1142–1152. *https://doi.org/10.1542/peds.2008-1862*

CONCLUSION

RAISING HEALTHY, RESILIENT KIDS

YOU'VE ALREADY STARTED

On a Tuesday evening, Sarah is on her couch, reading this chapter on her phone. Her seven-year-old, Connor, had a tough day. He got in trouble at school for pushing another child at recess, came home upset, threw down his backpack, and yelled, "I hate school! Everyone is mean to me!"

Her first reaction was to lecture him, ground him, or try to fix things quickly. But she chose not to.

She paused, got down to his level, and said, "Connor, I see you're really mad right now. That sounds like a really hard day. I'm here. Let's sit together for a minute." His shoulders relaxed, and the tension in his body eased. After five minutes together on the couch, he shared the whole story: another child had been teasing him all week, and he finally lost his temper.

Sarah listened and acknowledged his feelings, but didn't excuse his actions. They discussed what he could do differently next time. She called the teacher, made sure there was a consequence, and supported him throughout.

That night before bed, Connor said something she would always remember: "Mom, thanks for not yelling at me today. It helped."

That's what this book is about.

Not perfection. **Connection.**

Along with connection, there's another key idea from every chapter: your child's immune and nervous systems aren't fragile like glass. They are living systems, more like a muscle or a library than a vase. They grow through practice, stress, and recovery. Every infection, fever, or meltdown isn't a sign you've failed; it's another "book" in their immune library and another practice round for their emotions.

A resilient child is not one who never gets sick or never struggles. A resilient child is one who gets sick, gets care, and gets back to play; who feels big feelings, gets support, and learns they can move through them.

WHAT YOU NOW KNOW

If you've made it to the end, you know something many parents don't: resilience, both immune and emotional, is built over time. It's not just luck or a fixed trait. It grows day by day through experiences and your relationship with your child.

You now know:

- Your child's immune system is adaptive, not broken. It needs exposure, practice, and recovery to build its "library" of responses.
- Your child's nervous system is adaptive, not broken. When they act out, they are coping with stress, not failing at being "good."
- Toxic stress is real and measurable, but so is the protective power of one caring adult—and that adult is often you.
- Sleep, good food, movement, stress relief, and a supportive home are the main things that help your child's immunity more than any pill or supplement.

- Modeling matters more than lecturing. Your child learns how to handle frustration, illness, and setbacks by watching how you handle yours.
- Validation comes before correction. Whether it's a tantrum or a fever that cancels plans, naming the feeling comes first; the plan can come next.
- Praising effort and process ("You worked so hard on that," "You listened to your body and rested") builds resilience; praising outcomes alone builds fragility.
- Boundaries aren't mean; they're the frame that helps children feel safe in their bodies, their routines, and their relationships.

These aren't just ideas—they're real tools. And you're already putting them into practice.

The "Big Rocks" (So You Don't Have to Remember Everything)

You won't remember every vitamin D dose, humidity level, or supplement detail. During tough weeks, focus on a few key habits you can rely on.

1. Sleep is the base layer.

Getting enough sleep is the foundation for your child's immune health, learning, and mood. Protect bedtime, lower screen time, and keep routines simple. This helps their immune system more than any fancy remedy.

2. Food as daily medicine.

You don't need to ban treats. Cutting back on added sugar and adding more colorful fruits, vegetables, and whole foods helps the gut, where much of immunity begins. Aim for "one more color on the plate," not perfection.

3. **Movement as immune circulation.**

Active play and time outside keep the immune system working and help release stress. Even ten minutes of "floor is lava," jumping, or playing in the yard makes a difference.

4. **Connection as a stress buffer.**

Stress, conflict, and loneliness can make kids more likely to get sick or have meltdowns. Regular hugs, silly moments, and relaxed check-ins help calm their nervous system and give their immune system a better foundation.

5. **Trusting your gut.**

If you feel something isn't right with your child, trust your instincts. Asking for help isn't overreacting—it's working together with your pediatrician.

6. **Natural first, when it's safe.**

When your child is sick, begin with the basics you've built: rest, fluids, simple home remedies, good food, and a healthy environment. Medicines are important when needed, but they don't have to be your first or only option.

The details in this book are important, but when you're tired, focus on sleep, food, movement, connection, and a home that helps your child heal. These are what matter most.

YOUR 30-DAY RESILIENCE CHALLENGE

You don't need to try every strategy in this book right away. In fact, doing everything at once is the quickest way to burn out.

Instead, choose one thing.

Pick one strategy that feels meaningful and doable right now:

- A 10–15 minute daily check-in: a few minutes of focused, low-key connection.
- "Validation first": before correcting behavior or solving the problem, name and validate the emotion.
- Effort-based praise: shifting from "You're so smart" to "I saw how hard you worked on that."
- A repair practice: apologizing honestly when you mess up, every single time.
- One immune habit: protecting bedtime, adding one veggie a day, or starting a simple after-school "shoes off, wash hands, change clothes" routine.

Practice that one strategy every day for 30 days.

- Week 1: It feels awkward and easy to forget. Keep going.
- Week 2: It feels slightly more natural. You notice small shifts in your child. Keep going.
- Week 3: You catch yourself doing it automatically. New pathways are forming—for both of you. Keep going.
- Week 4: It feels like second nature. Your child responds differently because you're showing up differently.

Once that first strategy feels natural, add a second one. Slow, steady change is the kind that lasts.

When You Mess Up (And You Will)

You will yell when you meant to stay calm.

You will minimize a feeling when you meant to validate.

You will push through a day you meant to protect as a "rest day."

This isn't failure. It's just part of being human.

What matters is what you do next: the repair, the apology, the reset.

"I'm sorry I yelled. I was feeling stressed, and that was my problem, not yours. I'm working on handling my big feelings better."

That's the real lesson. It's not about being perfect, but about making things right.

Your child doesn't need a perfect parent. They need a real one—someone who makes mistakes, admits them, and keeps trying. That teaches emotional and immune resilience better than any script or supplement ever could.

Whole-Family Resilience and the Ripple Effect

Raising resilient kids isn't something you do alone. It takes the whole family learning together—parents, caregivers, and kids all slowly changing habits around food, sleep, stress, screens, and school routines.

As your kids grow, they become more independent, spending time with friends, joining teams, and trying new things. They'll eat snacks, stay up too late, and follow their peers. Your job isn't to stop every mistake, but to build a strong foundation of knowledge, experience, and trust. That way, when they do make mistakes, they'll return to you and the healthy habits you've taught them.

And the work doesn't stop with them. When you raise a resilient child, you're raising someone who will:

- Navigate friendships with empathy instead of cruelty.
- Handle illness and setbacks without spiraling into shame.

- Manage stress without relying only on self-destructive coping.
- Build healthier relationships instead of repeating harmful patterns.
- Show up for their own children someday with the same steadiness you're practicing now.

You're not just helping your child through this winter's illnesses or this year's school problems. You're shaping how they—and the next generation—will handle tough times. This work matters. It's your legacy.

For the Parent Who Feels Like It's Too Late

If you're thinking, "But I've already messed up so much," this part is for you.

I know you may feel guilty, replaying moments in your mind and worrying that you've done lasting harm to your child.

It is not too late.

Your child's brain is still developing. Their immune system is still building its library. Their nervous system is still learning what safety feels like. Their capacity for resilience is still being built.

What matters most for your child's resilience isn't your past mistakes. It's how present you are with them now.

If you've yelled, dismissed feelings, overcorrected, pushed too hard, or missed early signs of illness—welcome. This book is for you. The fact that you're reading, thinking, and trying to improve means you're already the parent your child needs.

You are enough. You always have been.

THREE QUIET COMMITMENTS

As you finish this book and return to the real, sometimes messy world of parenting, think about making three simple promises—not to me, but to your child and yourself:

1. I will show up.

I promise to be present, even when it's tough. I'll protect the basics—sleep, meals, check-ins, and rest days—so my child's immune and nervous systems feel safe and supported. I won't do it perfectly, but I'll do it consistently.

2. I will repair.

When I lose my temper or miss a sign, I'll come back, apologize, and try again. I'll show my child how to handle mistakes and recover with kindness, and that relationships can survive conflict because love is stronger than imperfection.

3. I will remember the why.

On tough days, I'll remind myself that I'm not just managing behavior or filling out school forms. I'm helping my child learn to handle sickness, disappointment, and big feelings—and come out stronger and wiser.

I am building resilience. That's some of the most important work there is.

ONE LAST STORY (AND A BLESSING FOR THE ROAD)

Six months after that Tuesday night, Sarah received a call from Connor's teacher. Her heart dropped. She thought, "Not again."

But the teacher wasn't calling to complain. She was calling to share something remarkable.

That morning, another student had been crying at his desk after struggling with a math problem. Without prompting, Connor walked over, knelt, and said, "It's okay to feel frustrated. Math is hard. I'm here if you want help."

The teacher said she had never seen a seven-year-old show so much emotional intelligence and empathy. Sarah hung up and cried—not because Connor was perfect, but because she saw he was learning, taking in, and sharing the secure base she had built for him.

That is what resilience looks like.

As you finish this book, remember this:

- The bedtime routine you protect when you're exhausted.
- The calm voice you choose when you want to shout.
- The apology you offer after you lose your cool.
- The validation you give instead of the lecture.
- The day you let your child stay home and rest instead of powering through.

These aren't small things. They are the building blocks for your child's lifelong ability to handle challenges, manage emotions, and heal.

You're not just getting through parenthood. You're building resilience—immune, emotional, and relational.

You're already doing it.

Keep going. The world needs the resilient kids you're raising.

And your child needs you, just as you are: imperfect, trying, and showing up.

That's enough. It always has been.

Bonus 1

Parents' Cold & Flu Checklist

This section is your "It's 2 a.m., and I can't think" guide—a quick reference for the nights when a child suddenly wakes up hot, coughing, or miserable.

Quick-Action Checklist: "They Just Woke Up Sick"

In the first hour, focus on:

- Check the temperature.
    - o Under 3 months old and 100.4°F (rectal) or higher → go to the ER immediately.
    - o Older than 3 months → note the number, but pay even more attention to how your child looks and acts.
- Hydrate.
    - o Offer a small sip of water, coconut water, breast milk, or formula right away. Tiny, frequent sips matter more than one big drink.
- Cancel and clear the schedule.
    - o As soon as you reasonably can, let school, daycare, coaches, or caregivers know your child is sick. Give yourself and your child permission to pivot to "rest mode" instead of trying to push through.
- Start your "acute protocol" (if approved by your provider).
    - o This may include zinc, vitamin C, elderberry, probiotics, or other supports you and your child's

clinician have already discussed. Having a simple written plan on the fridge can help you act without overthinking.

- Humidify the air.
    - Turn on the cool-mist humidifier in your child's room to keep nasal passages from drying out and to ease coughs.

Emergency Tips for Busy Families

These are small systems you can set up on calmer days, so you're not scrambling on the hard ones.

- The "Sick Bin."

Keep a clearly labeled bin in an easy-to-reach spot stocked with: tissues, a working thermometer (with extra batteries), vomit bags or an old towel, hand sanitizer, and a dosing chart from your child's provider.

- The "Tag-Team" Plan.

Before the next illness hits, talk through a basic plan:

- Which caregiver stays home on which day if a child is sick?
- Who can cover nights if there's more than one sick kid?
- The Batch-Cook Backup.

On a weekend when you have a bit of energy, make an extra batch of chicken soup or bone broth and freeze it. Label it clearly as "sick-day soup" so it's ready when a child can only manage a few spoonfuls of something warm.

- Over-the-counter cold medications: Should explicitly warn that these should not be used in children younger than 4 years due to potential harm and no proven benefit

RED FLAG SYMPTOMS

While most childhood illnesses are minor, it is vital to know the "red flag" symptoms that require immediate medical attention. Seek urgent or emergency care right away for signs like serious trouble breathing, blue or gray lips/face, confusion, or a rash that does not fade when pressed. Trust your instincts—if your child is extremely lethargic, severely dehydrated, or you feel that something is seriously "off," do not hesitate to call your pediatrician or go to the nearest emergency room.

FEVER REDUCER INSTRUCTIONS FOR INFANTS (BIRTH TO 12 MONTHS)

Section	**Acetaminophen (Tylenol)**	**Ibuprofen (Advil, Motrin)**
When to use	Can be given to babies 2 months and older with your doctor's approval.	Only for babies 6 months and older. Do not give to babies under 6 months. Do not give if your baby is dehydrated or not drinking well.
Dosing	Give 10–15 mg per kilogram (mg/kg) of your baby's weight every 4–6 hours. Maximum: 4 doses in 24 hours. Never exceed 75 mg/kg total in one day for infants.	Give 5–10 mg per kilogram (mg/kg) of your baby's weight every 6–8 hours. Maximum: 3–4 doses in 24 hours. Never exceed 30–40 mg/kg total in one day.

Section	Acetaminophen (Tylenol)	Ibuprofen (Advil, Motrin)
How to give	- Weigh your baby (use weight, not age, to calculate the dose). - Use the measuring syringe that comes with the medicine—never use a kitchen spoon. - Give by mouth when possible (easier to control the dose than rectal). - Wait at least 4 hours between doses.	- Weigh your baby. - Shake the bottle well. - Use only the measuring device that comes with the medicine. - Give with food or milk if it upsets your baby's stomach. - Wait at least 6 hours between doses.

Important safety rules

- Never give both medicines at the same time or switch back and forth between them.
- Never give aspirin to children—it can cause serious illness.
- Check all medicines your baby is taking to make sure they don't already contain acetaminophen or ibuprofen.
- Keep a written record of what medicine you gave, how much, and when.
- Remember: Fever itself is not dangerous—it's the body's way of fighting infection. You don't need to treat every fever; only when your baby seems uncomfortable.

When to call the doctor right away

- Any fever in a baby under 3 months old.

- Fever over 104°F (40°C) at any age.
- Your baby won't drink or is showing signs of dehydration.
- Fever lasts more than 3 days.
- Your baby is very sleepy, floppy, or hard to wake up.
- Rash appears with the fever.
- Your baby is crying and you can't comfort them.

Bonus 2

Immune-Boosting Recipes

Food is one of the most loving and practical ways to support your child's immune system. These recipes are designed to be nutrient-dense and kid-friendly. They tie back to the "rainbow," "power sprinkle," and "no-naked-carb" ideas from Chapter 4.

1. The "Traffic Light" Smoothie (Vitamin C Boost)

A fun way to get red, yellow, and green into one cup.

Ingredients

- ½ cup frozen strawberries (red)
- ½ cup mango chunks (yellow)
- 1 handful baby spinach (green—call it "Hulk Juice" or "Monster Slime")
- ½ orange, peeled
- 1 cup coconut water (hydration base)
- 1 teaspoon honey (optional, for kids over 1 year)

Method

- Blend on high until completely smooth. Serve right away.

Why it helps

- Strawberries and oranges bring vitamin C; spinach adds magnesium and folate; coconut water provides natural electrolytes.

2. "MAGIC MINERAL" CHICKEN NOODLE SOUP

A classic comfort food upgraded with immune-supportive herbs.

Ingredients

- 4–6 cups bone broth (chicken or beef)
- 2 carrots, sliced
- 2 celery stalks, chopped
- 1 cup cooked chicken, shredded
- 1 cup egg noodles (or rice for gluten-free)
- 2 cloves garlic, minced
- 1 inch fresh ginger, grated
- ½ teaspoon turmeric powder
- Salt and pepper to taste

Method

- Simmer carrots and celery in the broth until tender. In the last 5 minutes, add garlic, ginger, and turmeric so they stay fragrant and potent. Stir in cooked chicken and noodles just long enough to warm through.

Why it helps

- Garlic has natural antimicrobial properties; ginger supports digestion and can ease nausea; turmeric has anti-inflammatory properties that can soothe when kids feel achy.

3. Zinc-Rich "Power Seeds" Trail Mix

A lunchbox-friendly way to support zinc intake.

Ingredients

- 1 cup pumpkin seeds (pepitas)
- ½ cup sunflower seeds
- ½ cup dried cranberries or cherries
- ¼ cup dark chocolate chips (around 70% cocoa)

Method

- Mix everything in a jar. Scoop a small portion into snack containers for the week.

Why it helps

- Pumpkin seeds are one of the richest plant sources of zinc; dried fruit adds vitamin C and sweetness; dark chocolate brings antioxidants.

APPENDIX A

"SUPER KID" DAILY DEFENSE CHART

DAILY HABIT	**MON**	**TUE**	**WED**	**THU**	**FRI**	**SAT**	**SUN**
RISE: Drank water 💧	[ ]	[ ]	[ ]	[ ]	[ ]	[ ]	[ ]
FUEL: Ate a fruit or veggie 🍎	[ ]	[ ]	[ ]	[ ]	[ ]	[ ]	[ ]
MOVE: Played outside or jumped 🏃	[ ]	[ ]	[ ]	[ ]	[ ]	[ ]	[ ]
REST: Screens off 1 hour before bed 😴	[ ]	[ ]	[ ]	[ ]	[ ]	[ ]	[ ]
CALM: Breathing or cuddle time 🤗	[ ]	[ ]	[ ]	[ ]	[ ]	[ ]	[ ]

You can print this chart and put it on the fridge. Let your child check boxes or add stickers. It turns healthy habits into a simple game, not a lecture. You don't have to check every box every day; the visual reminder simply keeps the big rocks in sight.

APPENDIX B

DOSAGE CARD TEMPLATE

Keep this card inside your medicine cabinet and update it after pediatric visits so you're not doing math at 2 a.m.

CHILD'S NAME: ____________________________________

CURRENT WEIGHT: ________ lbs / ________ kg

DATE UPDATED: ________________________

MEDICATION	STRENGTH (from bottle)	MY CHILD'S DOSE (ml or tsp)
Acetaminophen (Tylenol)	160 mg/5 ml	________ ml
Ibuprofen (Motrin)	100 mg/5 ml	________ ml
Vitamin D3	________ IU/drop	________ drops

Safety reminder: Always double-check the concentration printed on the bottle before dosing, especially when you buy a new brand or bottle. Ask your child's clinician to help you fill this out and update it as your child grows.

APPENDIX C

WHEN TO CALL YOUR PEDIATRICIAN FOR COLD AND FLU

Common Cold and Flu Symptoms

Runny or stuffy nose, cough, sore throat, fever, body aches, headache, and fatigue are all common. Most kids recover at home with rest and fluids, but some symptoms deserve a call or a visit.

Call your pediatrician if your child has:

- Fever lasting more than 3 days, or a fever that returns after going away
- Any fever in an infant under 3 months
- Trouble breathing, fast breathing, wheezing, or pulling in at the ribs
- A cough lasting more than 2–3 weeks
- Ear pain, drainage from the ear, or a very severe sore throat
- Vomiting or diarrhea that is not improving, or signs of dehydration (dry mouth, no tears, less urine)
- Poor feeding or refusal to drink
- Extreme fatigue, unusual weakness, or difficulty waking
- Symptoms that are getting worse instead of better after 5–7 days
- Flu-like symptoms in a child with chronic conditions (like asthma, heart disease, or immune problems)

Seek urgent or emergency care right away if your child has:

- Serious trouble breathing, blue or gray lips/face, or pauses in breathing
- No urine for 8–12 hours in an infant, or 12–24 hours in an older child
- Confusion, severe headache with stiff neck, or a seizure
- A rash that does not fade when you press on it
- Severe or persistent chest pain
- Signs of severe flu complications (cannot walk because of muscle pain, very high fever that won't settle, or sudden worsening after starting to get better)

Home Care Basics

- Offer fluids often and encourage rest.
- Use fever reducers as directed for your child's age and weight.
- Use saline, a humidifier, and gentle suction (for infants) for nasal congestion.
- Keep your child home from school or daycare until they have been fever-free for 24 hours without medicine.

Key takeaway: Trust your instincts. If your child doesn't look or act like themselves, or if something feels "off" to you, call your pediatrician. You are the expert on your child; this book and your medical team are here to support you.

APPENDIX D

NATURAL REMEDIES AND SUPPLEMENTS —WHAT WE REALLY KNOW

These are the gentle, home-based tools we've returned to throughout the book. Use them as options, not obligations, and always follow your child's provider's guidance.

Symptom	**"Kitchen Cure"**	**The Strategy**
Sore throat	Dark honey (buckwheat, etc.)	1 teaspoon straight or in warm water for kids over 1 year. Coats and soothes.
Ear pain	Garlic/mullein oil	Warm the bottle in your hand; 2–3 drops in the ear **only if** there's no drainage and no tubes.
Stuffy nose	"Steam tent"	Sit with your child in a steamy bathroom for 10–15 minutes before bed to loosen mucus.
Fever >102°F	Tepid bath or "wet socks."	Use lukewarm water to cool gently; avoid cold baths—wet-sock trick to draw heat down toward the feet.
Nausea	Ginger tea/ice chips	Very small sips over time. Avoid heavy foods. Let the stomach rest.

Safety considerations

- Regulation: Herbal products are not FDA-regulated; quality and purity vary
- Contamination: Heavy metals, pesticides, and adulterants have been found
- Interactions: Herbal remedies can interact with conventional medications
- Adverse effects: Underreported; clinicians should monitor closely

Clinical guidelines and expert recommendations

- AAP guidance: Counsel families on risks, benefits, and evidence; monitor for adverse effects
- Risk–benefit framework: Use when considering CAM therapies
- Communication: Discuss all therapies openly to avoid interactions and ensure safety

Conclusion and recommendations

Natural remedies and supplements have limited evidence; some have modest benefits, but safety and quality concerns persist. Clinicians should:

- Prioritize evidence-based conventional therapies.
- Use a risk–benefit approach for CAM
- Counsel on product quality, dosing, and monitoring
- Maintain open communication about all therapies

Overall, most natural remedies and supplements lack strong pediatric evidence; use caution, prioritize safety, and base decisions on the best available evidence.

REFERENCES

Probiotics for the prevention of pediatric antibiotic-associated diarrhea. (2011). The Cochrane Database of Systematic Reviews. https://pubmed.ncbi.nlm.nih.gov/22071814/#cabfad64

Vitamin D for the prevention of disease: an endocrine society clinical practice guideline. (2024). The Journal of Clinical Endocrinology and Metabolism. https://academic.oup.com/jcem/advance-article/doi/10.1210/clinem/dgae290/7685305?login=false#3d5d36b5

The evidence base for complementary medicine in children: a critical overview of systematic reviews. (2011). Archives of Disease in Childhood. https://pubmed.ncbi.nlm.nih.gov/20605859#6a8a7a59

Pediatric integrative medicine. (2017). Pediatrics. http://pediatrics.aappublications.org/content/early/2017/08/24/peds.2017-1961#6acf3d06

Zinc for prevention and treatment of the common cold. (2024). The Cochrane Database of Systematic Reviews. https://www.cochranelibrary.com/cdsr/doi/10.1002/14651858.CD014914.pub2/full#4d326b19

Herbal medications (...). (2016). JAMA. https://jamanetwork.com/journals/jama/fullarticle/2499278#0f714715

Complementary and alternative medical therapies for children with cancer. (2004). European Journal of Cancer. https://pubmed.ncbi.nlm.nih.gov/15341976#9936dc41

AUTHOR BIO

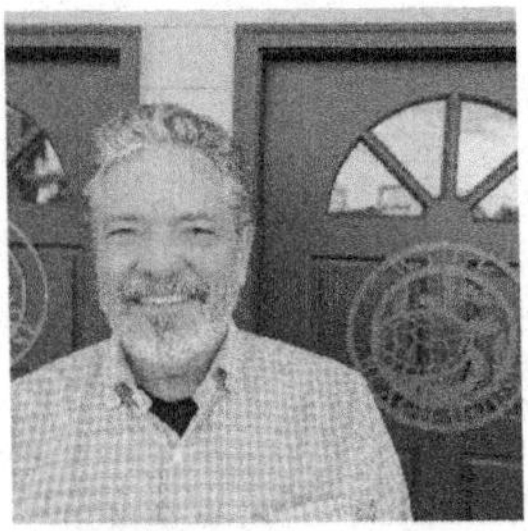

Michael J. Vicioso, CPNP-PC, is a pediatric nurse practitioner dedicated to supporting children's health and well-being through evidence-based, family-centered care. With a professional focus on pediatric development and preventive health, he works closely with families to provide practical guidance that supports healthy growth from infancy through childhood.

Through his clinical work and educational initiatives, Michael is committed to empowering parents with clear, accessible information they can trust. His approach emphasizes collaboration, education, and compassionate care, helping families navigate everyday health concerns with confidence.

Professional Moniker
Michael J. Vicioso, CPNP-PC

Official Website
www.ghtkids.com

QR Code
A QR code has been generated that links directly to the official website:
www.ghtkids.com

NOTES

This document consolidates the currently available official author information and links for internal reference and publication preparation.

Made in the USA
Coppell, TX
07 May 2026

76754190R00085